Keeping Promises
Georgia Stories

Gillian Russell Grable

INSTITUTE ON HUMAN DEVELOPMENT AND DISABILTIY / UCEDD
UNIVERSITY OF GEORGIA
COLLEGE OF FAMILY AND CONSUMER SCIENCES

I want to sincerely thank the families featured in this book who graciously invited me into their homes and shared the intimate details of their lives. May all families always find the support of people close to their hearts to help them fulfill their promises to each other.

Author: Gillian Russell Grable
Graphic Design: Rebecca Brightwell
Cover: *Everyday Heroes* Quilt by Beth Mount, PhD

Institute on
Human Development
and Disability

a unit of

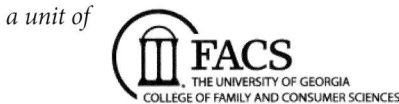

© 2014 University of Georgia
Institute on Human Development and Disability

A University Center for Excellence in Developmental
Disabilities Education, Research and Service (UCEDD)

A Unit of the College of Family and Consumer Sciences
www.ihdd.uga.edu
706-542-3457
info@ihdd.uga.edu

Produced under grant number 90DD0562 from the U.S. Department of Health and Human Services, Administration on Developmental Disabilities.

CONTENTS

Chapter One   Ethel and Belinda: A Promise   4

Chapter Two   Who Will be There for My Susannah?   14

Chapter Three   David Thompson, A Christian Man   22

Chapter Four   Taking Care of Aunt Sarah   30
I Just Thought That's What People Did

Chapter Five   I Promised Eddie I Wouldn't Send Him to a Nursing Home   38

Chapter Six   Used to Go to Church Sharp as a Tack   46

Chapter Seven   I Always Measured My Boyfriends by How They Reacted to Jimmy   54

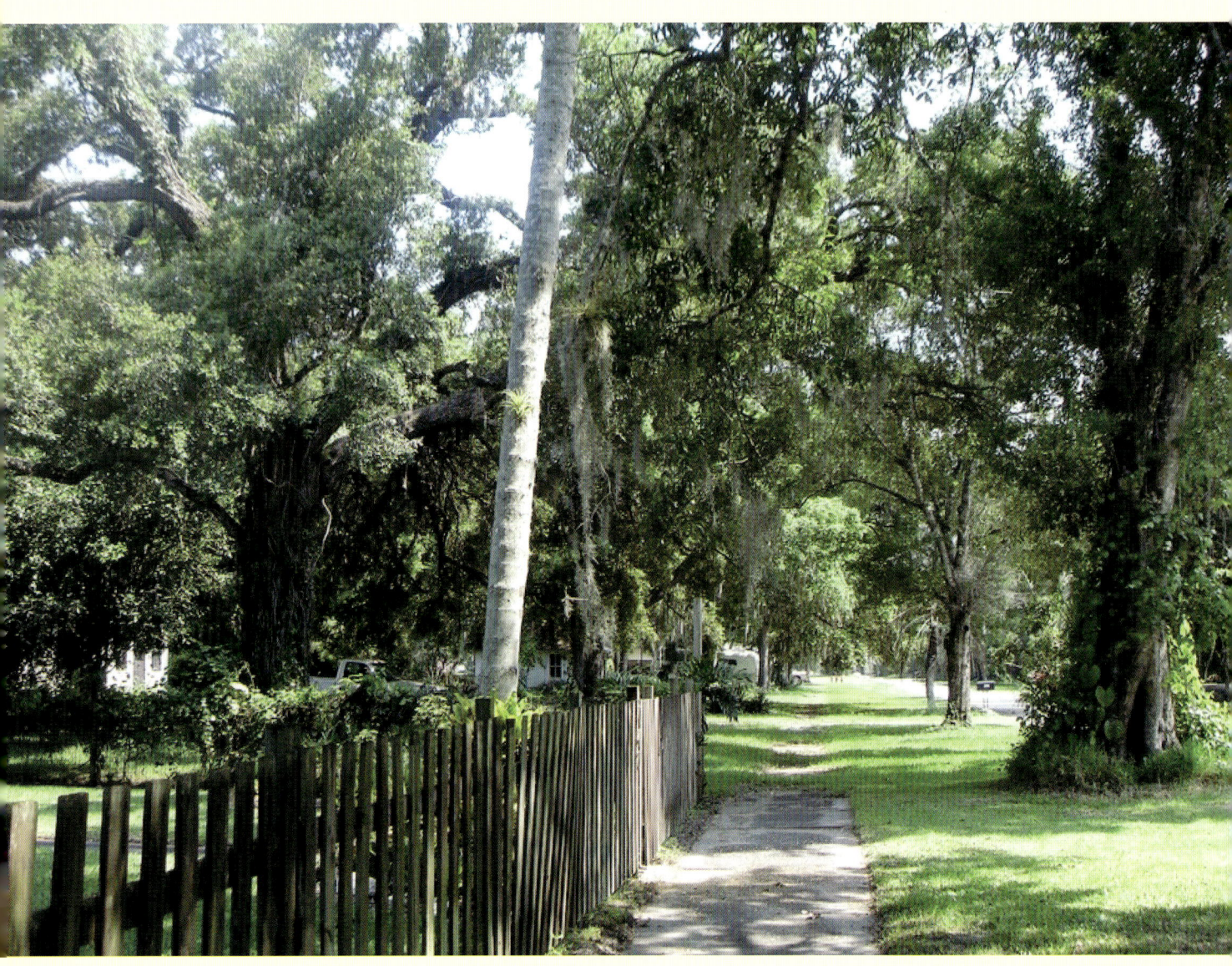

Names and identifying details have been changed to honor the privacy of the family.

Chapter One
Ethel and Belinda: A Promise

Driving east on Georgia Highway 22 past lavender wisteria vines draping the dark green leaves of magnolia trees, a deer leaps across the highway to join another on the side of the road. I see signs for "Meehaw Jelly" and the "Anytime Beauty Salon" as I slow down for the sign saying, "Deerville City Limits." I pass a young man sitting in the back of a pick-up truck ready to begin the day's work, and turn off Main Street onto Mockingbird Lane. As I walk up to the faded yellow house with a tin roof covered in pollen, Belinda, a 61-year-old woman with soft brown skin, watches me through the screen door.

We walk down the hallway dividing the rooms of the house into a large room with dark red curtains drawn. The bright sunlight through the curtains is enough to reveal a couch, a chair, a television, and some boxes. Belinda lies back in her chair and begins her story:

"I work from 7:00 to 7:00 in a factory standing all night on a concrete floor. I try to sleep after I get off before Ethel comes home from the center.

"My mother and Ethel's mother were first cousins; when Ethel's mother died, Ethel moved in with my mother. I promised my mother to keep her when she died. I just took the role and stepped into my mother's shoes. Didn't nobody else step up to the plate to get her, so I just followed what my mother followed. Ethel's been with me seven years.

"I promised my mother to keep [Ethel] when she died. I just took the role and stepped into my mother's shoes."

"I was about 12 years old when I got to know my cousin; Ethel was 26 then and dressed real nice when we went to Trinity CME together. My mother and Ethel's mother were on the usher board. They are buried behind the church. I can still hear the hymns 'Swing Low Sweet Chariot' and 'What a Friend We Have in Jesus.' Her mother's house is still standing. Ethel used to rake their yard real good with a dogwood broom, and she would have the house spotless. She went to a training center then -- I don't know what they taught her."

Ethel, a young-looking 75-year-old woman, walks slowly into the room leaning on her cane, her light brown face framed by a short black wig. The dark circles under her soft brown eyes light up as she describes living with her mother:

"My mamma, she was a good cook -- collards, pintos, turnips, and potato pies. Helped her cook and pushed the buggy when we shopped for groceries. Remember my mother reading the Bible aloud to me.

"I loved swinging on the porch together in front of the big floor fan. I can smell the chicken frying and taste the dinner -- butter beans, tomatoes, squash and okra. We had 20 chickens -- I used to collect the eggs in a pan. We used to give them to people in the neighborhood. Oh -- we used to bake: Pineapple upside down cake, bread pudding, and home homemade biscuits."

Ethel and Belinda's grandmothers lived in a time when quilt frames were draped over chairs in the living room. Ethel remembers, "Grandmother wouldn't let me help her with the quilts -- treated me like a child. I toted the water from the well to the house. Scrubbed the clothes on the washboard. I helped pick the collards, turnip greens, tomatoes. We had rose bushes and Easter lilies. Horace, my brother, and me, we used to play in the dirt making mud cakes. Horace, he passed away."

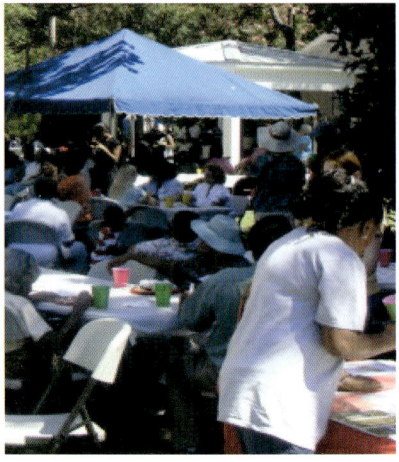

"I can smell the chicken frying and taste the dinner — butter beans, tomatoes, squash, and okra."

Ethel and Belinda: A Promise   6

Belinda, looking at Ethel, exhaustion in her eyes, says, "I've been organizing my family reunions for ten years. Ethel goes with me. We have a fish fry and a banquet. Sometimes we have them in state parks. We go to the festival here in late October. Ethel's relatives come around, but they mostly talk with me. Ethel has a nephew who used to come and take her home with him for the weekend, but he's only come twice this year. Ethel lived with an aunt in Ohio for almost a year a while back.

"We stay in church all day Sunday. I get the spirit there -- if it makes me cry I know the Lord has touched me. I love to hear 'It's Me, It's Me, It's Me Oh Lord, Standing in the Need of Prayer.' I'm stuck in the middle – my son has problems. Taking care of Ethel has taken a toll on my personal life – I just don't have anytime for myself. She talks to herself a lot.

"I'm studying for my associate degree so I can work with children when I retire. My friend has a personal care home – I'll give Ethel to her next year. Her doctor at the mental health center said Ethel would get worse the older she gets. I keep telling her, 'You don't want to go across that bridge.' " (The regional psychiatric hospital lies across the river.)

The road about a mile west from Deerville meanders through pine forest on one side and fields fenced in with rusted barbed wire on the other. Crossing a very bumpy wooden bridge over the railroad tracks below, Ethel rides a van on this road every day at 9:00 AM to the new Senior Center, which sits alone on the left in the middle of a field. Ethel and the other ladies and gentlemen, 25 in all, enter the main room filled with folding tables and chairs. They pass walls decorated with construction paper Easter bunnies and chicks. Ethel, dressed in a light yellow pantsuit, puts her purse in a chair and goes to the coffee maker to pour a cup for herself and her friend, Mildred, who is 88 years old. Sitting down next to Mildred, who is

"We stay in church all day Sunday. I get the spirit there — if it makes me cry I know the Lord has touched me."

reading the newspaper, Ethel describes the activities of the center: "Some play pitty-pat or spades -- most exciting thing is TV. Long time ago had arts and crafts. Sometimes we exercise in chairs. Once they let us sew on the sewing machines, but the teacher left. See this sunflower I glued on my purse? Isn't it pretty?"

Mildred peers over her glasses, puts down the newspaper, and picks up the conversation, saying, "This is the only recreation we have, coming here. When we were younger we all used to do domestic work or keep children -- that is all of us except Ethel. I've been knowing some of these folks here all my life. My sister and brother come here. We used to have lots of stores in Deerville. Churches used to have bake sales on Main Street. I read about stuff in our weekly paper -- they had a community picnic last year, but I didn't go. Didn't have a way."

As if a bell had rung, Ethel jumps up at 11:00 AM, washes her hands with hand sanitizer, goes to the counter in front of the kitchen, and brings a box to the table. She begins to put white paper placemats in front of each person and lay a package of plastic utensils, as if they were silverware, to the right of each placemat. At 11:15, the gentleman sitting behind Ethel says the blessing, and everyone is served chicken and vegetables on Styrofoam plates.

[One month later. I have introduced Ethel to Jane and Frances, citizens of Deerville who want to see their community thrive. We are visiting Jane's home.]

The smell of freshly mown grass fills the air as Ethel carefully cuts the old blossoms on vibrant red roses next to the porch of Jane's antebellum home. "Looks good Ethel, helping those new blooms grow. Did you know if we dried the rose hips we could make tea?" Jane says to Ethel, as she digs nearby, transplanting irises. Ethel lifts her head and beams at Jane. Jane, a petite woman with short gray hair, explains,

"When my husband and I moved to Deerville and bought this old house, I wanted to be able to welcome the community. Come on up for some iced tea Ethel -- Frances is here." As Ethel takes her seat on the porch at the round wicker table set with three glasses of iced tea, Frances greets Ethel. "I'm glad to see you, Ethel," she says. "What do you think about making a pineapple upside down cake for the community potluck?" Frances, her hair adorned in braids, puts her arms around Ethel for a warm hug as they sit together with Jane.

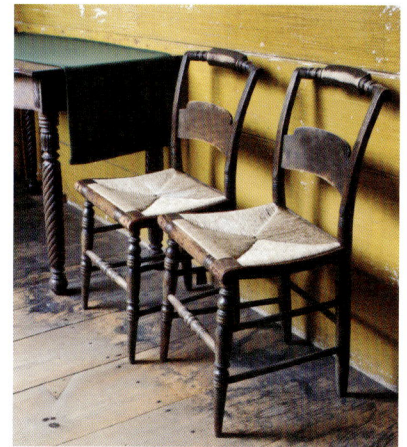

The three women drink iced tea and plan the second annual community potluck to be held in August on the lawn surrounding Jane's house. "Do you think your church would lend us some folding tables Ethel? Last year we had enough the churches loaned us, to seat four hundred people," Jane says with dancing blue eyes. Frances describes with excitement in her voice, "Oh, we had a fine gathering. Mr. and Mrs. Reynolds came -- did you know, Ethel, they've owned the hardware store on Main Street for 37 years? And Officer Katherine came-- she grew up here as a little girl and moved away. But she's been back now a couple of years working in the police department. I just have the feeling the days when Main Street was filled with shops, is coming back. Did you know a hundred years ago Deerville was a stage coach stop and had one of the best hotels in Georgia?"

The clear brown eyes of Frances meet those of Jane and Ethel. "I'd love to show Ethel your antique chair collection, Jane. Can we go downstairs?" As Frances and Jane help steady Ethel on her cane down several stairs, a small door underneath the porch reveals several rooms with stone walls. One long room with 50 small chairs, some caned, some with leather seats, seem lined up as if school is about to begin. The three women cross the hallway and enter the former billiard room, with dark wood paneling. They sit on several antique chairs next to a small fireplace . . . one can imagine the stories told a hundred years ago from these chairs.

Ethel and Belinda: A Promise

Ethel, picking up doll furniture resting on the table, remises, "I used to make doll furniture like this, with popsicle sticks at the training center. Don't make anything anymore."

The three women talk about Deerville and how to bring some celebrations of who the people are to their town. Frances describes her longing, saying, "A local woman wrote several plays a few years ago and produced them at the high school -- a hundred people came. What talent!"

Sitting in the chairs talking, Jane begins to tell the story of how she and her husband planted three acres of organic garden around their home: "I love the smell of the oregano, parsley, basil as I walk through the rows of onions bulging out of the earth." Then Ethel describes going to the well for her grandmother. Frances says, "I was told that too -- get to the well before dark or you'll get a whupping."

The three women tell more stories and toss around some ideas for a celebration. Frances exclaims, "I got it! The church nearby -- the pastor's been clear he wants to help. We can have something like 'strolling down memory lane': everyone can share their story and have an ice cream social at the church on a hot summer day." Jane and Ethel nod with enthusiasm.

Frances' face leans closer to Jane and Ethel. "I want to tell the fable of 'Stone Soup' at our church ice cream social . . ."

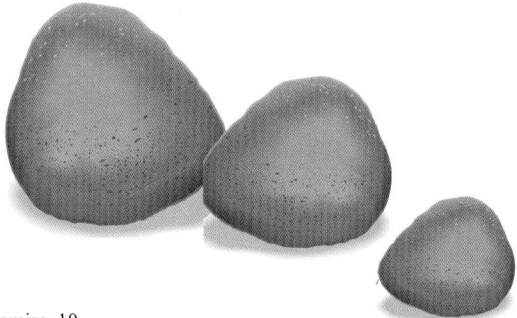

Stone Soup

Once upon a time, there was a great famine upon the land. Three soldiers, hungry and weary of battle, came upon a small and impoverished village. The villagers, suffering a meager harvest and fatigued from the many years of war, saw the three soldiers come upon them. Quickly they hid from sight what little they had to eat.

They met up with the three at the village square. "There's not a bite to eat in the whole province," they told the soldiers. "You'd better just keep moving on to the next village."

"Oh, but we have everything we need," one soldier said. "In fact, we were thinking of making some stone soup to share with all of you. You, sir, look hungry. Would you like some?"

"Stone soup! What a ridiculous thing!" the villagers exclaimed. "You can't make soup from a stone!"

But the three soldiers gingerly reached into their pockets, and each of them in turn slowly pulled out a smooth, round stone. They inspected their stones closely and nodded to one another in assent. "We have brought with us some wonderful stones that should make for a great and hearty soup. Do you have a large cauldron we might borrow to make our stone soup?"

Overcome with hunger and unable to feed the guests staying at his inn, the local innkeeper was intrigued with the idea of making soup from stones. With help from the soldiers, he pulled a large iron cauldron from the kitchen of his inn and placed it in the center of the village square. The three soldiers filled it with water, and built a roaring fire under it.

Then, with great ceremony, the three soldiers took the three stones they had collected on their travels and placed them into the water one at a time. They waited for their stone soup to come to a boil, stirring occasionally with a large wooden spoon.

"Do you know what would really help this soup?" asked one of the soldiers. "A hefty dash of salt and pepper! You can't have a good stone soup without salt and pepper, after all."

Timidly, one of the villagers said, "Well, I think might be able to find some salt and pepper that have you might have, if I can share in your stone soup!"

The soldiers quickly nodded and assured the villager that there would be plenty of stone soup to go around, with such a large cauldron of soup on the boil.

By now, hearing the rumor of food, most of the villagers had come to the square or were watching the events of the village square attentively from their windows. As the soldiers fastidiously stirred and sniffed at the "broth," they licked their lips in anticipation. The hunger of the villagers began to abate their initial skepticism.

"Ah," one of the soldiers said rather loudly, "I do like a tasty stone soup. Of course, stone soup with cabbage is hard to beat."

"Oh, yes," added another soldier, "Cabbage really adds flavor to stone soup."

After a few moments, a villager approached hesitantly, holding a cabbage he'd retrieved from its hiding place, and added it to the pot.

Another villager came up and inspected the pot and said, "You know, I have some carrots. That would really add flavor and color to this soup, too!" He ran off to his home to fetch the colorful vegetable.

"Yes, yes, this will be a fine soup," said the third soldier; "but a pinch of some parsley would really make it a soup fit for a king!"

Up jumped a villager, crying, "What luck! I've just remembered where some has been left!" And off she ran, returning with an apron full of parsley and with a turnip, too.

As the kettle boiled on, the memory of the village improved. In short time, barley, salted beef and rich cream had found their way into the great pot. A grand keg of beer was rolled into the square as the entire village sat down to a great feast. They all ate and danced and sang well into the night, refreshed by the feast and delighting in their newfound friends.

In the morning, the three soldiers awoke to find the entire village standing before them. At their feet lay a satchel filled with the village's best breads and cheeses.

"You have given us the greatest of gifts: The secret of how to make soup from stones," said an elder. "Rest assured that this is something that we shall never forget and that we shall forever cherish."

The third soldier turned to the crowd, and said: "Whereas there may be no real secret to stone soup, one thing is certain: It takes many and all to make great feast." And with this, the soldiers kindly accepted their satchel of breads and cheeses and went on their way, never to return.

It is said that soon after meeting these soldiers, the village quickly returned to its former prosperity, and has thrived ever since. The soldiers are said to still walk from town to town collecting stones along the way, and sharing their secret recipe for their famous stone soup.

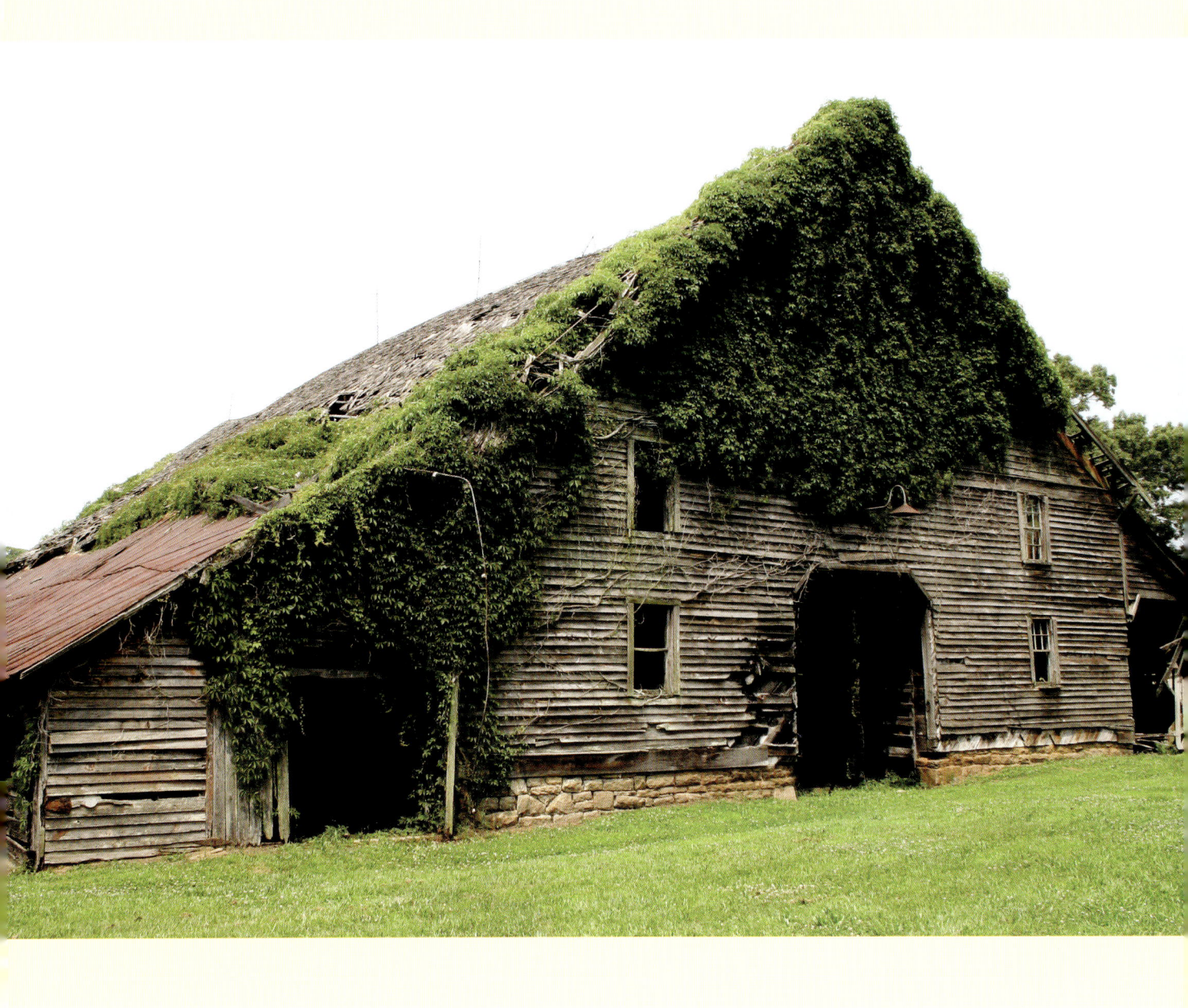

Chapter Two
Who Will Be There For My Susannah?

Driving north from Atlanta I cross the Chattahoochee River and turn onto a parkway leading me into Cherokee County. Along the roadside is a mixture of new subdivisions and abandoned weathered wooden homes, one reinforced with metal Coca Cola signs nailed to the sides. A horse peacefully grazes in a field nearby, and the morning light touches the magnolias busting with flowers. Just after passing a barn covered like a bedspread with kudzu vines, I turn into the subdivision where Susannah lives.

Susannah's dad, Sam, a spry 71-year old-man, welcomes me into their stucco home, where they have lived for 11 years. A wooden clock in the shape of a gable with a glass door sits on the mantle piece. "I grew up with that clock," Sam says. "My Daddy paid $100 for it in 1947. We were so proud of it on the mantle in our home. It still runs. That clock is almost as old as I am," he laughs with ease.

He introduces his oldest daughter, Susannah, 44 years old, and her younger brother, Adam, 39 years old. Susannah, who wears a very short brown hairstyle, watches with curiosity as Adam describes them growing up:

"I remember Halloween," he says. "My older brother, John, was dressed as a cowboy, I was Superman, and Susannah was an Indian with long braids.

"Susannah was 10 that year, and on her birthday, my brother, John, told her, 'Susannah you're 10 now. You can ride your bicycle.' John

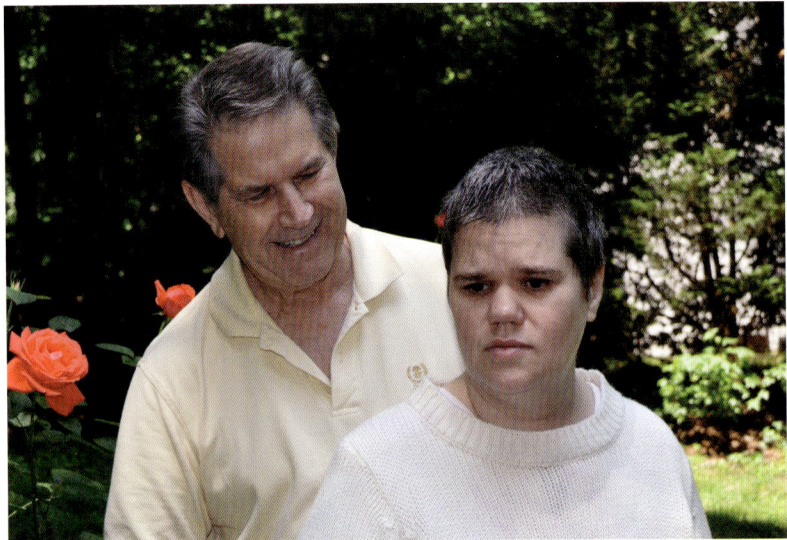

Sam and Susannah

took the training wheels off, and Susannah sailed around the cul-de-sac where we lived."

"I think I was a little scared," Susannah says shyly.

Then Adam, a slender man with his long hair pulled back, looks fondly at his sister and calls forth one memory after another:

"When I played with Susannah it was always with her horses, -- hundreds of toy horses. She used to write the most wonderful stories about ponies -- 'Little Pony' is the one I remember the best. We moved to Canton where Dad raised about 25 horses on 60 acres. Susannah and I used to ride Petite -- she was the most gentle horse we had.

 "On the horse farm, we used to get up real early with Momma, all three of us and Dad too, and pick blackberries along the driveway. I remember us carrying straw baskets and the jelly Mamma made.

She dripped the syrup over the pot as the blackberries were bubbling and could tell when it was just right. She had to make sure she had the right mixture of red and black berries to get the pectin just so.

"We used to sit at the kitchen table, I think it had a flowered linen tablecloth, and watch Momma cook. Her meringue cookies had chocolate candy kisses in the middle – they were out of this world. And at Christmas time her plum pudding . . ."

"It was really something else," Susannah finishes Adam's thought. Susannah opens a spiral notebook, one of many where she has written recipes for desserts like "Mocha Log" and "Chocolate Surprise." She leafs through another notebook where she has made lists of subjects: "Art, 1st favorite, Math and Spelling, 2nd favorite, Trigonometry and Physiology." One notebook lists all the holidays imaginable including New Year's Eve Day and National Milkshake Day. Another notebook lists the names of her favorite stores and restaurants.

"When I sold the horse farm, we moved to Forsyth County," Sam continues. "Susannah graduated from high school right there with the whole graduating class. When they called her name all one hundred and fifty kids stood up and cheered. I was so happy," Sam recalls with a quiver in his voice.

"When Susannah was born she seemed to be a perfect baby, but my wife had contracted measles while she was pregnant. Susannah has always spoken in a halting way; before she turned four years old she entered special education. They told us she would reach a certain age and not progress beyond that, but I refused to believe it. I taught her how to ride – that was not difficult. No problem with a bicycle – she caught onto that real quickly. My wife was an avid reader, and Susannah acquired her reading skills from her. She can read most any word.

"Susannah is a really good singer -- she loves country western music and gospel; anything with a fast beat to it. She can listen to a song once or twice and pick up the words. We went to charismatic churches. When Susannah was very little she would go to the children's Sunday school and was really good at memorizing the Bible. We used to go to church with some friends Linda and Cecil -- Cecil is very outgoing, and Susannah always looked for him at church to get a big hug. We are a very affectionate family.

"Susannah worked at the training center after high school for fifteen years," he continues. "They put labels on boxes. On weekends they would go to movies and dances. Susannah had a good friend, Doug --- they fell in love."

Susannah's dark brown eyes light up and a smile crosses her lips as she says, "We were sweethearts. Doug gave me a red rose, and he said it meant true love. I believe it."

"My wife wanted to be near the beach, so we moved to St. Simons in 1998," says Sam. "Susannah went to the training center there. She cut scrim for fishing traps. Susannah made good money there, a couple of hundred a week. She was real good at cutting the scrim to a certain size. We enjoyed ourselves at the beach. Kyle, Susannah, my wife, and I rode bikes a lot."

"I took the lead family bicycling," Susannah remembers, looking to her father for reassurance about her memory. "Mother and I used to draw pictures and paint. She was a great artist. I draw pictures of people and animals, especially horses running."

A family photo from St. Simons sits in a gold frame on the top of the upright piano in the living room. Everyone is dressed for dinner in the photo: Susannah in a beautiful white dress, stockings, and shoes with her father, mother, and her brother, Kyle.

"When we moved back to Alpharetta from St. Simons," Sam continues, "my wife wasn't feeling well and Susannah didn't go back to a center. For four years we searched for the source of my wife's illness. Adam, my middle son, moved back to help me take care of Susannah when my wife was bedridden.

"Six years ago we all knew that my wife was going to die. Susannah seemed to accept it, but she knows death is a window. She believes that we will see her again, but there is a void that takes a long time to accept.

"Not long ago we had a conversation at the kitchen table -- me, Susannah, her younger brothers, Adam and Kyle. We were celebrating a birthday and talking about how much my wife loved celebrations. We all cried. That's the only time I remember Susannah crying. She and her mother were always hugging each other -- her mother became very sick for a very long time -- Susannah would sit in her room and talk to her. She died while I was reading 1 Corinthians 13.

"We didn't go to church for a while. By then my youngest son Kyle, was having some difficulty at school – I had to home school him. I had all I could handle after my wife died. I needed to reorganize my life and get back on track. That's when I contacted SOURCE; Susannah's caseworker told me about personal care homes. I took Susannah to visit a home in Dahlonega in 2006, and she liked it. She used to read the Bible to her roommate.

"I brought Susannah home from Dahlonega after some months because she complained about her stomach hurting so. We had every kind of test imaginable done and couldn't find anything. I would wake up in the middle of the night to see Susannah standing at the end of my bed crying. My wife's illness was so similar I just wonder how closely related Susannah's complaints were. 'You know I am saved, I am not afraid to die', Susannah would tell me.

1 Corinthians 13 (NIV)

[4]Love is patient, love is kind. It does not envy, it does not boast, it is not proud. [5]It is not rude, it is not self-seeking, it is not easily angered, it keeps no record of wrongs. [6]Love does not delight in evil but rejoices with the truth. [7]It always protects, always trusts, always hopes, always perseveres.

[8]Love never fails...

[13]And now these three remain: faith, hope and love. But the greatest of these is love.

"I needed someone here with Susannah while I was working. Otherwise I wouldn't have been able to work to get the income I needed.

"Susannah told me around this time that she wanted to go back to work. She wanted to work with children – she loves to have babies in her lap. I contacted the training center and they asked me if she had a waiver. I didn't know what they were talking about. I applied for the NOW waiver, and they told me they didn't have any money; she is on the waiting list."

Susannah sits next to a collection of shells underneath a glass side table that she picked up on the beach when they lived in St. Simons. She looks at her father. "I like to work and get paid – just like cutting the scrim at the training center. I like to buy presents.

"Clover helps me buy presents for the animals for Christmas," Susannah explains, smiling at the young woman seated nearby. Clover has been Susannah's paid companion (through SOURCE) for seven months now. Since she has known Clover, Susannah's stomach pains have lessened. Clover comes 40 hours a week to be with Susannah. Clover smiles. "Susannah is a pleasure – she has a great sense of humor," she says. "We have a lot of fun together."

"We were notified by SOURCE in December 2009 that Susannah's services would be terminated, but that it would take a while. Two weeks later I got another call letting me know the services would be terminated within a couple of weeks. The caseworker said we could appeal it, and they suggested I contact legal aide. We ended up going to court – the judge ordered the services to be reinstated, and that was October 2010. The judge gave both sides two months to work it out.

"We lost SOURCE for several months -- Adam and I took turns staying with Susannah. If Susannah is left at home by herself, she can't use the telephone, and one day she turned on the burner under a plastic bowl. They have continued to temporarily reinstate services every couple of months. I expect we will loose our SOURCE services eventually.

"Even if I live to be 90, I won't be able to take care of Susannah then -- I will need someone to take care of me. But who will be there for my Susannah after I am gone? Kyle and Adam love Susannah; Adam said to me, 'I would die for her.' I told him, 'You have got to live for her.' I can imagine her living in a family environment with Adam or Kyle. They would need some help during the day, and if they got married, figuring out how Susannah could still be a part of the family. Susannah belongs in the family -- she is family." Susannah nods her head and smiles as she opens one of her notebooks to read a story she has written...

On the Ranch and in the Mountains

Illustration and Story by Susannah

Once upon a time we lived on a ranch with horses. There was a yellow baby horse that was wild. Her name was Goldie. There were also many black and brown horses that were also wild. Goldie was my favorite. She was so beautiful. There was also a tame horse that the cowboy rode. The tame horse Sunshine and the cowboy Sam used to go off to the mountains all the time. One day they came up on a bear that tried to chase them. That bear was so slow; they thought it must have been part turtle. After that they came up on a turtle. That turtle ran up to them so fast they didn't know what to think. That turtle bit Sunshine right on the ankles. They were sure that turtle had to be part bear. Sunshine and Sam decided the mountains were just too crazy. They went home and never went back.

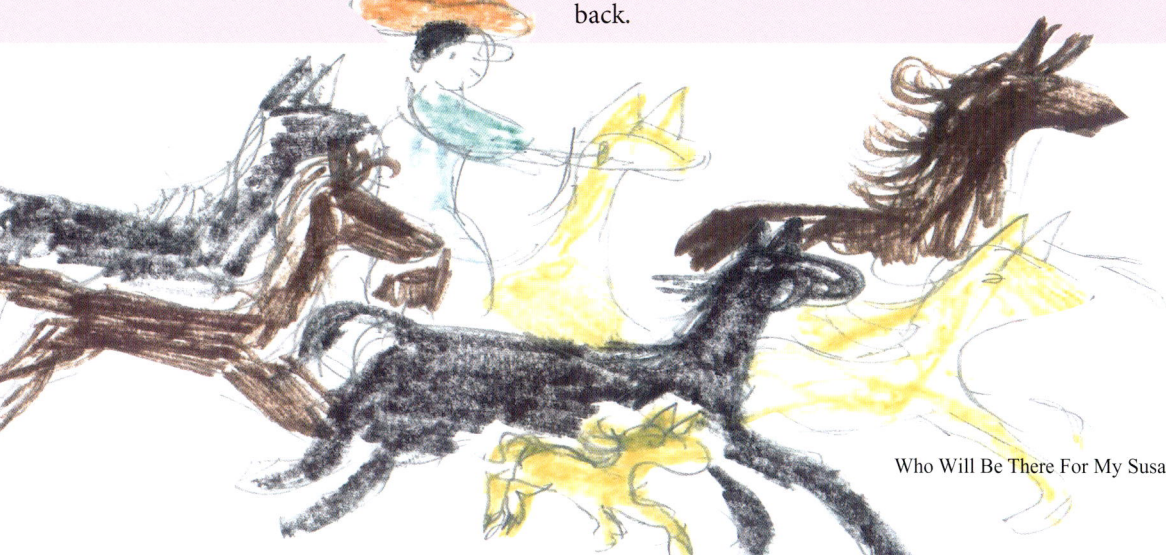

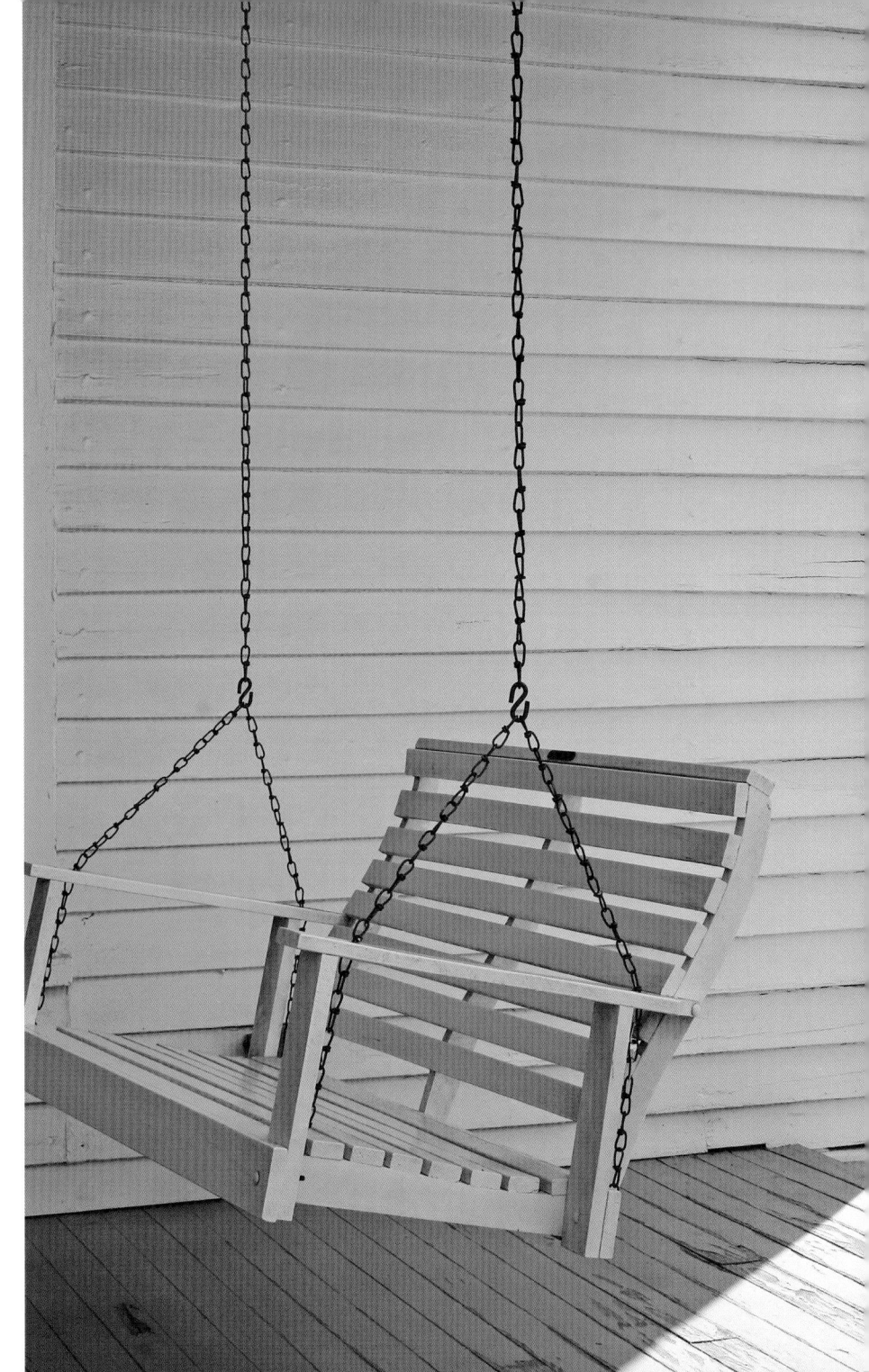

Names and identifying details have been changed to honor the privacy of the family.

Chapter Three

David Thompson, A Christian Man

Driving southwest from Cordele on State Route 300, I see groves of magnificent pecan trees. I leave the highway and travel through town until I see a weathered steel mailbox with lettering, "D W Thompson."

The screen door on the porch creaks as I open it. I pass the wooden swinging chair and wonder how many summers this porch has heard the soft voices of conversation on a hot evening. The chime of an antique clock beckons me into the house. A sign on the front door says, "Don't count the day done until you've made the day count."

Marguerite Thompson, petite with silver-white hair, sits next to several visitors and greets me as I enter. She feels a little tired from the dialysis she takes three times a week, but her voice is strong.

"I was born in Alabama on December 1, 1921," she says. "My grandfather had been a sharecropper. My mama was forty-two when she had me; I was the youngest of ten children! We grew up building fires, washing dishes, making candy and cookies to give to friends. She taught me how to cook a potato salad right."

Marguerite moved to Georgia in sixth grade when her daddy sold their farm. After graduating from high school, she worked in a children's clothing store for 19 years and then as a teacher's aide while raising her family of four children: Stephen, Arthur, Carol, and David. 23 years ago, Marguerite moved to south Georgia to be close

"Don't count the day done until you've made the day count."

to her daughter, Carol, and get help with taking care of her husband who had Alzheimer's disease.

David, her youngest son, now 49 years old, was named after his daddy. Marguerite recollects, "So many difficulties. Stephen was two when my husband was in World War II. Arthur, Carol, and David came after Stephen. Carol moved to south Georgia, and Stephen died in 1972. Arthur lived to be 64 years old before he died. If you don't have bad luck, you don't know what a blessing is."

The clock chimes at 3:30 PM as David walks through the door, returning from his day at a sheltered workshop. A dapper man with graying hair, David gives Marguerite a kiss on the cheek and sits down at the upright piano in the corner of the living room. "Sweet Hour of Prayer" fills the house. "When he was little," Marguerite says, "David took piano lessons for two weeks. The teacher told me, 'I can't teach him -- he wants to play by ear.' Do you know that when he walked up to the stage to play for the graduation exercises at the high school, a family behind me snickered. When I turned around at the end of the graduation to look at them, they were crying. I offered them my sympathy."

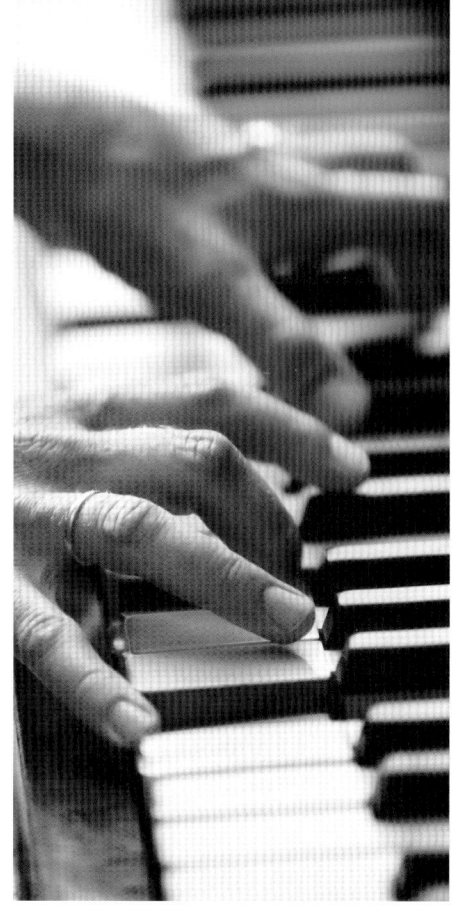

David worked for three days a week in a factory cleaning, but the plant closed after six months. He went on to a job cleaning at a local television station for six months and finally landed a job sweeping at a Christian bookstore five days a week for seven years. Then the bookstore was sold, and David returned to the sheltered workshop.

"David is very mechanical -- he loves to fix things around the house. He makes sure all the doors are locked at night and the alarm is turned on," Marguerite proudly describes of her only living son.

Marguerite's daughter, Carol, moved in 10 months ago to help Marguerite with getting to her dialysis treatments. On her way home from one trip to the dialysis center in February, her car hit a tree, and several weeks later Carol died. Carol's promise to her mother was that if something happened to Marguerite, she and David would live in the house together. Family members talked to Marguerite about plans they were making for her and David after Carol died. Marguerite told them she was not going to a nursing home and she and David were not going to be separated. "I went and looked at some of those nursing homes, but I am not as old as those people in there."

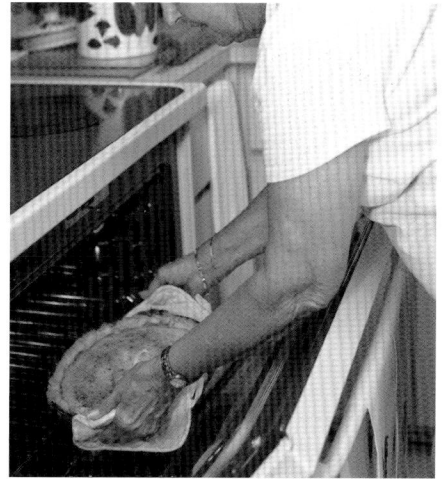

Since Carol's accident, Barbara has been coming to visit every day to cook and clean and listen. A neighbor for 23 years, Barbara met Marguerite while she was planting flowers in her front yard. Barbara's snow-white hair, pulled back in a ponytail, nods as she talks. "Marguerite would talk with the children I was caring for then, just like neighbors should," she says. "David and Arthur always looked good, and the lawn and house looked cared for. The value of this neighborhood -- Marguerite would cook on Sundays, and neighbors and church folks would fill the house.

"Ms. Denise, who runs the children's nursery, calls every day, and Ms. Turner brings eggs every week. She brings brown eggs for David. Frank stops by to see if there is something that needs to be fixed. And Ms. Rosalynn, the hairdresser, visits once a week. I have lived in this neighborhood for thirty years and I've met neighbors I didn't know through being here with Marguerite and David."

Through his steel-rimmed glasses, David's eyes soften. "My sister Carol was good to me -- she took me to the grocery store." He leans over and touches Barbara's shoulder with a quiet laugh, saying, "Barbara is a good friend too. My best friend Gertrude takes me to church -- Pastor Stanley preaches good."

Then Pastor Stanley's eager face and muscular arms gesture towards the family as he describes how he came to know Marguerite and David:

"I knew Marguerite's family even before I became a preacher," he says. Marguerite's family has always greeted us like life-long friends. Shortly after Arthur died they joined our church, and now everyone lights up when they see Marguerite and David come into church -- David takes to everyone. He laughs at my jokes and says 'Amen' when I make a good point. He even played 'Happy Birthday' for me on the piano.

"David was asked to join the Visitation Ministry; we visit people in nursing homes. David plays the old songs they love: 'The Old Rugged Cross', 'Amazing Grace,' and 'Oh How I Love Jesus.' If you name a song, David can play it."

"I feel happy when I'm playing music. I pray for people," David says and smiles.

"What makes David's day is going to church," says Marguerite. "Our friend Gertrude picks us up for Sunday morning, evening, and Wednesday evening service. When I can't go, David tells me where the preacher's sermon came from in the Bible. The Thompson family stands for church," she explains.

During Marguerite and David's years of welcoming people into their home, one imagines the grandfather clock in the corner of the living room chiming every 15 minutes. Marguerite slowly moves her walker over to the clock and eases down on her knees to find the date written inside. "December 1, 1974. My husband gave it to me for my birthday."

Opposite the grandfather clock is a wooden curio cabinet. Lit from behind, a glass angel with feathers gazes out on Marguerite and David and their home. Recently Marguerite fell while waiting for the ride to her dialysis appointment. "I managed to crawl over to my walker and pull myself up, but I cut my hand on the plate I was carrying," she says.

Pastor Stanley says the house is in need of many repairs, and with a $60,000 mortgage he wonders whether anyone would help fix it so that Marguerite and David could remain in their home. Marguerite's will needs to be changed so that the house is left to someone she trusts now that Carol has died. "We watch out for Marguerite and David," says the pastor. "We had to take action when family members were trying to move her out. Marguerite and David have rights from God. This is part of what our faith is."

Before Arthur died, his doctor was a man named Dr. Smith; he and his wife are devoted to making sure Marguerite and David remain together. Mrs. Smith is applying for spousal veteran's benefits for Marguerite; Dr. Smith has become her medical power of attorney. Marguerite and David are on a waiting list for an assisted living facility.

Barbara will ask several builders she knows to give estimates on what it would cost to renovate their home. She thinks there may be someone in the church community who would consider being a live in companion to David and Marguerite. Gertrude, who takes them to church, has become Marguerite's financial power of attorney.

The grandfather clock chimes as I say goodbye, and the door closes behind me. I see the pampas grass, nandina and camellia bushes surrounding the porch; a testament to Marguerite's many years of gardening. I see "D W Thompson" on the mailbox as I drive away, and know that David is now the man of this house.

[Two months later]

A small red brick church with a white steeple sits above State Route 300 facing a pecan grove. At 10:00 AM Sunday morning, cars are pulling in to park on the lawn in front of the church. The parishioners are greeted as they walk through the door and find their seats

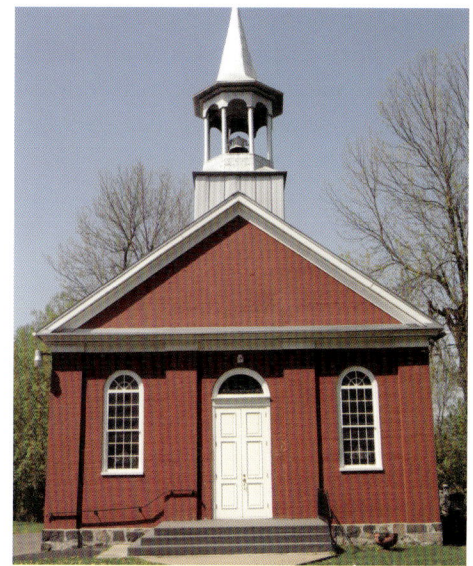

in one of the eight pews on either side of the church. Pastor Stanley's daughter is playing rousing music; her arms seem to bounce up and down on the piano keys as her foot pumps the pedal. Light beams through panes of lavender, gold, blue, and yellow windows. Members come to the front pew to hug Marguerite -- she smiles weakly and says she is so glad to see them. David, who has ridden to church with a friend, finds his mother, gives her a big kiss, and pulls her hand in his.

Marguerite's gnarled hand reveals a bandage from an IV line. She recounts, "My blood sugar got real low and they called the ambulance. They discharged me from the hospital to a nursing home -- one of my family advised me to go. I'd rather be somewhere else -- it's not me."

With the ceiling fan turning over his head, Pastor Stanley announces that the youth are dismissed for Sunday school. As the children leave their pews, two men come to help Marguerite into her wheelchair and back her down the stairs to visit the rest room before adult Sunday school begins.

Pastor Stanley preaches from the pulpit in front of a wooden table with a carved inscription: "This do in remembrance of me." A Bible lays open on the table in between two straw collection baskets. "What a beautiful day the Lord has prepared for us," says Pastor Stanley. "Teach us to learn what we need to know and help our leaders to make good decisions."

Marguerite returns to her pew and the pastor continues, "This year is the 400th anniversary of the King James Bible. Most of the Bible was written for hurting people and sojourners. How do we handle hurt and pain?" Marguerite's hand shakes as she finds the passages the pastor announces in her cloth-bound Bible. A napkin and pieces of paper mark certain pages.

Adult Sunday school ends, and Marguerite says softly, "It's a close-knit church." Her friend Gertrude, who acts as Marguerite's financial power of attorney, comes over to explain that she applied for Medicaid for Marguerite and hopes that there will be an alternative to living in the nursing home. David joins the conversation. "I'm happy in my new place," he says. "I take turns doing the laundry with my roommate. I bought a razor at the new discount store last week." *(Upon hearing that Marguerite was sent to a nursing home, Developmental Services requested emergency residential services for David and he moved into a duplex.)*

Barbara comments on what has happened to her neighbors: "I would love to see Marguerite be able to come back home -- she is a very self-willed person, but she doesn't seem to have a lot to say right now. The worst part is seeing Marguerite at her age almost as if she is forced into jail -- I cut some roses from her house and brought them to her last week. 'These are from your house Marguerite,' I said when I gave them to her. The lady visiting Marguerite at the same time as me said, 'Don't say that, she doesn't know she has a house.' Well Marguerite *does* know she had a home.

"Ms. Thompson has spent many years taking care of others -- her husband, her sons -- I never heard her complain. She had two children killed in an auto accidents and recently losing her daughter, then her home, and David has been hard on her. I can see her losing her will to carry on. I would live to see some loving person take her into their home -- she deserves to be pampered. I myself can't; I have an 86-year-old mother who needs my help. It would be great if she could be reunited with her son. We will miss them as neighbors.

"I almost didn't recognize David when I saw a group of people at the discount store the other day. I remember thinking, 'They must be from the sheltered workshop.' But I didn't recognize David -- Marguerite always made sure he was dressed neatly. I didn't recognize him as someone I knew."

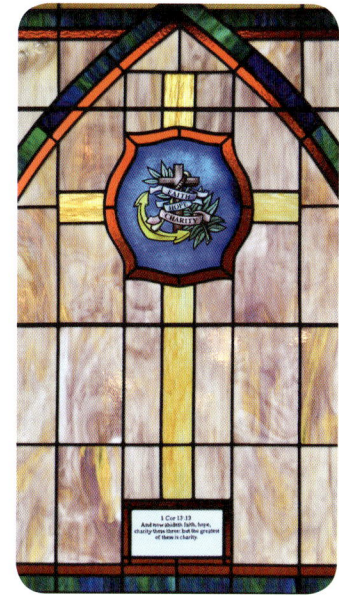

David Thompson, A Christian Man   29

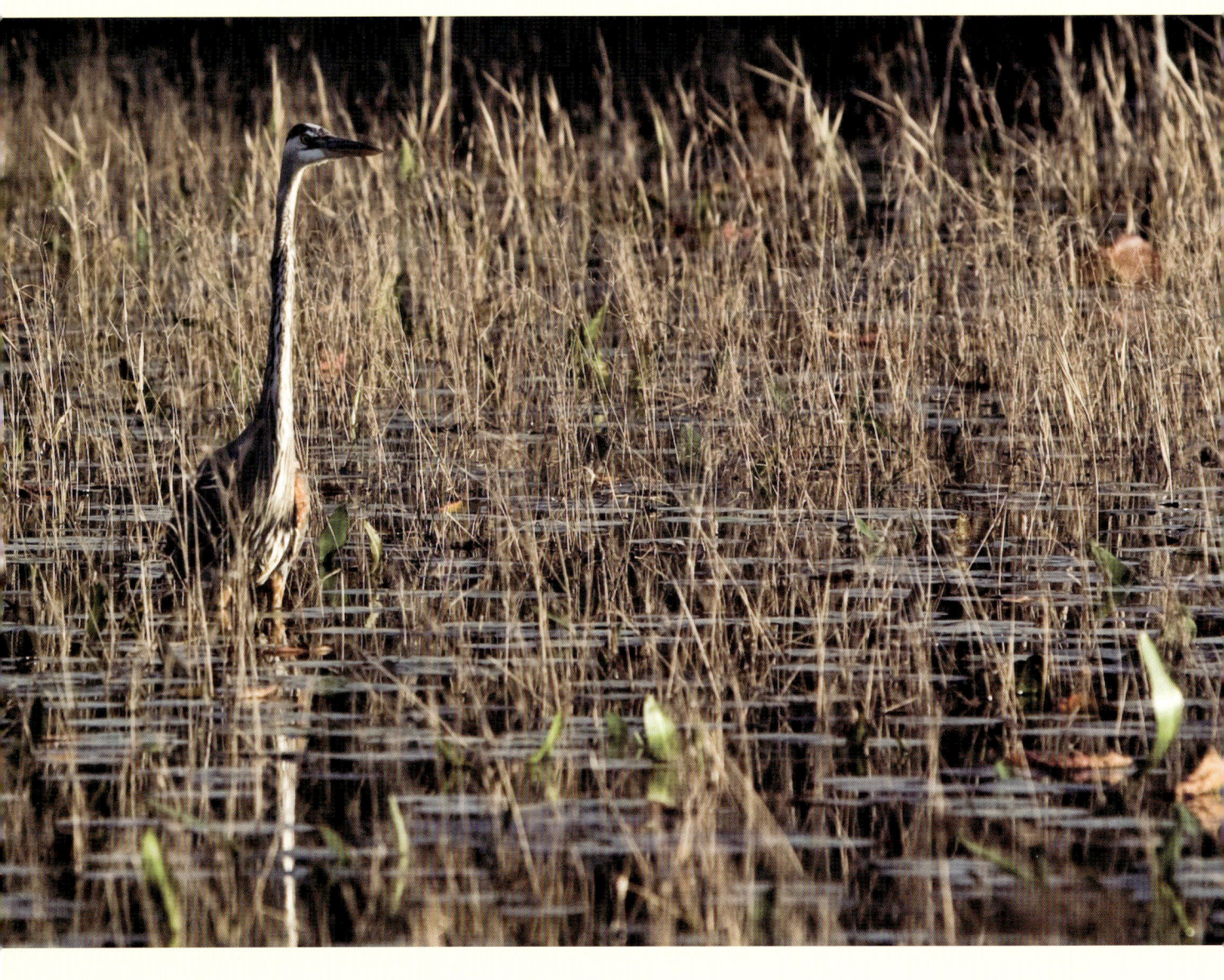

Chapter Four
Taking Care of Aunt Sarah
I Just Thought That's What People Did

Southbound US Highway 23 passes by short date palms and fields where tufts of cotton cling to the stalks after harvesting. There is a heron sitting in the middle of a pond just before the highway passes over the Ocmulgee River. Further down the highway, a sign announces, "Folkston: Gateway to the Okefenokee Swamp."

When I see the painted sign, "Philadelphia Free Will Church," I turn into the gravel road and drive past the pond to the top of the hill where Sarah's tin-roofed blue house sits. The sweet smell of wild pink honeysuckle enfolds me as I walk over the ramp to the front door. Sarah's petite, silver-haired 73-year-old mother, Robbie, welcomes me into the living room, every shelf and table top filled with pictures of her husband, four children, seven grandchildren, and fourteen great-grandchildren.

"Sarah is the youngest. She's 50, and I named her after my mother," Robbie says as she introduces me to her only daughter. Sarah, sitting in a blue recliner chair next to the window, greets me with an enthusiastic reach of her arms and dancing hazel eyes. "All the grandkids love their Great Aunt Sarah." Sarah beams listening to her mother's words, her arm resting on a colorful quilt.

Sebastian, nine years old with short black hair and eager eyes, looks across the room to Sarah. "If Aunt Sarah could speak, she would say, 'I have been waiting to talk. Happy to see you today.' That's what she's saying when she smiles."

Sebastian lives next door; he comes over every day at 6:30 AM. Robbie explains, "Sebastian wants to be the first one to turn the light on, give her a hug and crawl in bed with Sarah. This morning Sarah was massaging Sebastian's back with her feet."

Danny, Sebastian's grandfather, arrives every day soon after 6:30 and helps Robbie bathe and dress Sarah. Then Danny helps her walk into the living room and sit in the recliner. He and Robbie hook up the plastic tubing to a bag of nutrition that flows into Sarah's stomach. Robbie continues:

"Sarah has had a feeding tube for fourteen years. She had trouble all her life with food going into her lungs.

"For the first three years of Sarah's life, she was in the hospital about six times each year for aspiration. We said the Lord would help us because he gave her to us. When Sarah was about a year old, we took her to Gracewood in Augusta. They said she wouldn't live for six months, and if she did she would be nothing but a 'vegetable' and to leave her with them. I told them she was not a 'vegetable,' and if we were to put her in a place like Gracewood, our boys would be afraid that if they were sick we would put them away. I told them we would keep her.

"When Sarah was 10 years old we went to the Crippled Children's Center in Waycross where the staff of Gracewood came to see children in south Georgia. A doctor said, 'What have you done for her?' He could see Sarah was so smart on those matching tests. We hadn't done anything except what the Lord had done."

For the next 20 years, Robbie worked at the service center where Sarah spent her days. "You could tell the difference between the people who had stayed at home and those who had been sent away," Robbie says. "Those people returning from hospitals hadn't been introduced to as many things. They had been treated differently -- they weren't dressed right and didn't have manners."

About 7:45 AM, Danny, with his gray hair pulled back in a ponytail and a big beard, walks Sarah back to bed for a nap. Ms. Irma, Sarah's home health aide, helps her back into her recliner at 10:30 AM. Danny's hazel eyes behind his gold rimmed glasses gaze at Sarah as he reminisces:

"Pop, my brothers, Tommy, Gadson, and I used to take Sarah in the truck hunting. One of us would sit in the truck with Sarah watching. Oh, and we've gone to the Okefenokee Swamp, put in a 9.9 motor boat, put Sarah in her wheelchair in the boat and a pole in her hand. She caught warmouth fish, mudfish and jacks. Sarah put her hand over her face with a smile once as if to say, 'Oh my, catching that fish.'

"Our grandpa gave the land for Philadelphia Free Will Baptist Church right up the road from this house. We gave Mom and Pop their fiftieth anniversary party at the church -- two cakes, and Sarah greeted all the family with a huge grin. She was dressed real pretty with a red long-sleeved shirt with cross-stitch flowers. Clara May, Mama's sister in Alabama, gave them this grandfather clock for their anniversary."

As the clock in the living room chimes twice for 2:00 PM, Danny looks out the window with Sarah. "Daddy's been gone three years now," he says. "See the house next door? That's Uncle Newton's house. And you can tell when he's outside 'cause Sarah starts laughing.

"My wife Debra and I found out we have Choctaw and Cherokee heritage," Danny continues. "We take Sarah in April and October to the pow-wows at the tribal grounds in St. George. Everyone dances

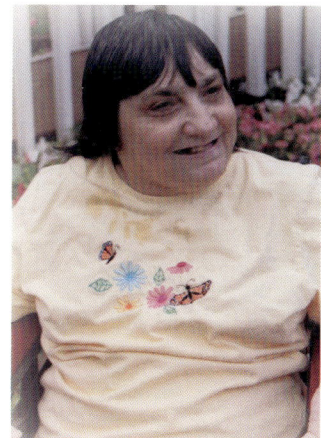

Sarah

Taking Care of Aunt Sarah   33

and we push Sarah, clapping around the arena. The tribal chief and his wife couldn't believe Mom and Pop had kept Sarah at home. They think the world of Sarah, so full of life and her knowledge of people and her surroundings. And Sarah loves to watch our grandson Sebastian dancing at the pow-wows."

Debra, with sad blue eyes and gray hair pulled back in a ponytail, begins to talk about her daughter, Bambi, and Sarah:

"When Bambi began to crawl as an infant, Sarah was about sixteen and scooting herself along the floor too. Bambi always wanted to sit in the chair with her Aunt Sarah. She had a special connection with Sarah; she could tell when Sarah was hurting.

"1992 I will never forget... Bambi was fifteen at the time, and they were all coming home from church one night. Bambi spent the night with Mom and Daddy in the trailer they lived in then. Seven people sleeping in the house and Daddy woke up as the fire started. Daddy broke a window, ran to the outside -- Mom handed Sarah through the window to him. Then Mom crawled through, went back in to get Bambi and the others, but she was knocked outside by an explosion.

"Robbie was in the hospital for three weeks for smoke inhalation. Sarah wouldn't eat or drink. I took her to my house and told her 'Mamma's okay.' When we had Bambi's funeral, Sarah cried the most heartbroken cry -- I never heard her like that."

Robbie started quilting several years after the fire and has finished quilts for her 14 grandchildren. She holds up the quilt underneath Sarah's arm for everyone to see the same pattern of cloth zigzags across -- a rail fence quilt.

"When we take Sarah to church," Robbie says, "she sings along with us, taps her foot, and holds the song book. She loves 'Amazing Grace'

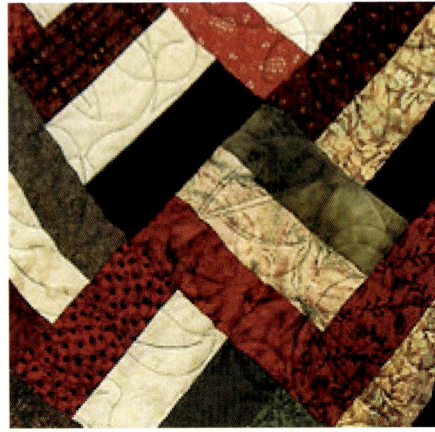

"Taking care of Aunt Sarah — I just thought that's what people did."

Taking Care of Aunt Sarah   34

and 'When We All Get to Heaven'. During testimony Sarah holds onto the back of the bench and the Lord knows what she is saying. The preacher says, 'God bless Sister Sarah!' If Brother Musgrove comes to visit us, Sarah puts her hand on his to ask him to pray for us. One time someone new from church came to visit us. 'Never seen anyone like Sarah. Don't know how to talk to her.' I told him to talk to her like anyone else. Now he calls and says, 'May I speak to Sarah?'

"When Sarah was a teenager, she was in the hospital in Decatur. Every time the staff tried to feed her she put her hands to her mouth. When I got there I folded my hands for grace with Sarah and then she ate. The staff finally realized she wouldn't eat before saying the blessing. Here at home at mealtime, Sarah holds her hands together while we say 'Amen.'

"Before the feeding tube, we used to go to church every Sunday morning and evening and Wednesday night. We could go more places before the tube; we used to walk to the highway and back -- about a mile. We still go to church dinners, but now she needs her feeding or water and medicine six times a day. Sarah gets breathing treatments four times a day. I guess if I had two people to help me feed and change Sarah we could get to church on Sunday."

Nathaniel, Sarah's nephew, a tall 27-year-old young man, walks into the living room. He is a pediatric nurse in Jacksonville, Florida. Nathaniel remembers, "Several times a year, Sarah went to the Folkston hospital across the street from my school. I was in seventh grade; after classes I would cross the street to help Granny feed Sarah. I would sit with Sarah in her hospital room if Granny had to go somewhere. We had to make sure her head was up all the time so she wouldn't choke. At night Granny and I would try to sleep in the other hospital bed. Papa Dan would come at 5:00 AM, and Granny would take me home so I could shower and change to get ready for school. Taking care of Aunt Sarah -- I just thought that's what people did.

"When people are sick everyone is stressed out," Nathaniel continues. "We were sleep deprived. The nurses helped us out a lot. I guess that's why I wanted to be a nurse. One time at work I apologized to a seven-year-old patient of mine for my cold hands. He said, 'Your hands are cold, but you have a warm heart.'"

Sarah is holding a laminated photograph of family members' hands clasped together that her niece made for her. "Hands of Love" is written at the top of the photograph. Robbie muses, "A lot of people ask me, 'Aren't you depressed?' Sarah won't let you be depressed. We still go on vacation to Alabama to visit my mother's family for the reunion every August. Sarah's been to the Okefenokee Festival. When the kids were young, we went camping at Devil's Elbow campground near St. Mary's River. We brought a couple of tents and rolled Sarah around."

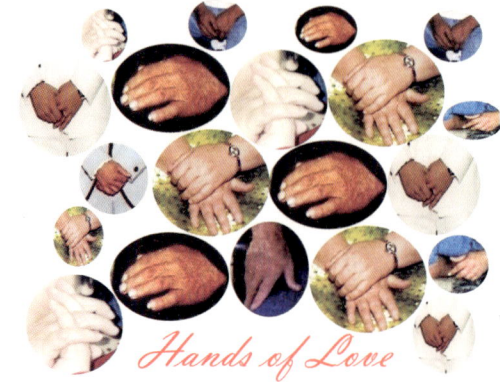

Gadson, Robbie's youngest son who lives with his mother and his sister Sarah, walks through the back door and joins the conversation. "I get off work every day about 3:30," he says, "so I'm here for the rest of the day. When we were young, Sarah went everywhere we went. If anyone had ever made fun of Sarah, they would have gotten punched.

"Long time ago," Gadson continues, "we went with Daddy to get a loan at the bank. Loan officer said, 'If I had a daughter like Sarah I wouldn't bring her out in public.' Daddy pulled the loan officer by his shirt across the table. 'Lord didn't see fit to give you a daughter like Sarah.' Daddy never went back to that bank.

Gadson's girlfriend Gail arrives and Sarah's grin widens. Gail explains, "When I visit, we always put Sarah in her wheelchair with my purse in her lap and wheel her to the back bedroom where Sarah puts my purse on the bed. Sarah wants me to take her to the bathroom to put clothes in the dirty clothes basket. She wants to work.

We put the folded clothes in her lap and push her down the hall to put them up."

Sarah looks at her wrist at about 4:45 PM. Robbie explains, "She used to have a watch but all the pins fell out. So now Sarah looks at her wrist to let us know it's time to eat."

Tommy, Robbie's middle son, comes by every day about 5:00 to help Robbie change Sarah and help her eat. When Sebastian and his brother get off their school bus, they come to visit with Great Aunt Sarah and help shake the bag to mix the nutrition with water.

Robbie reminisces about her middle son. "When Tommy was little," she says, "first thing he did when he got up in the morning would be to go to Sarah's crib and talk to her. I can still hear him saying, 'I love you. What are you doing this morning?' Sarah has always been right in the middle of all of it."

When Robbie passes, Sarah will remain in her home with Gadson. Debra has promised to take care of her. Tommy will become Sarah's legal guardian.

As I stand to give a farewell hug to Sarah and Robbie, Gadson shows me to door. I see rows of cabbages in the front yard he has planted behind red, yellow, purple, and white pansies. A warm wind is blowing from the gulf. I turn to wave goodbye to Sarah; she is looking out the window at the sparrows feeding on the bird feeder, but turns to give me a beautiful smile. Robbie stands at the door wearing her t-shirt that reads, "To know what love really means, you have to read between the lines."

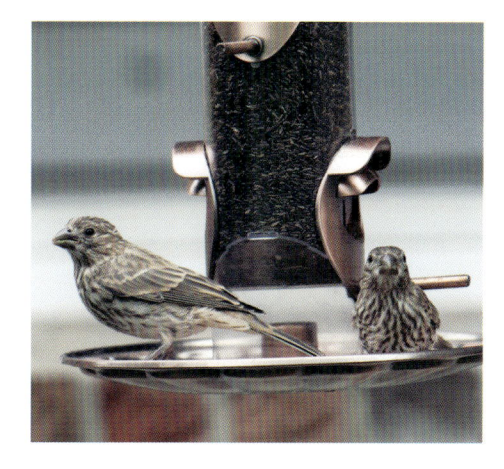

"To know what love really means, you have to read between the lines."

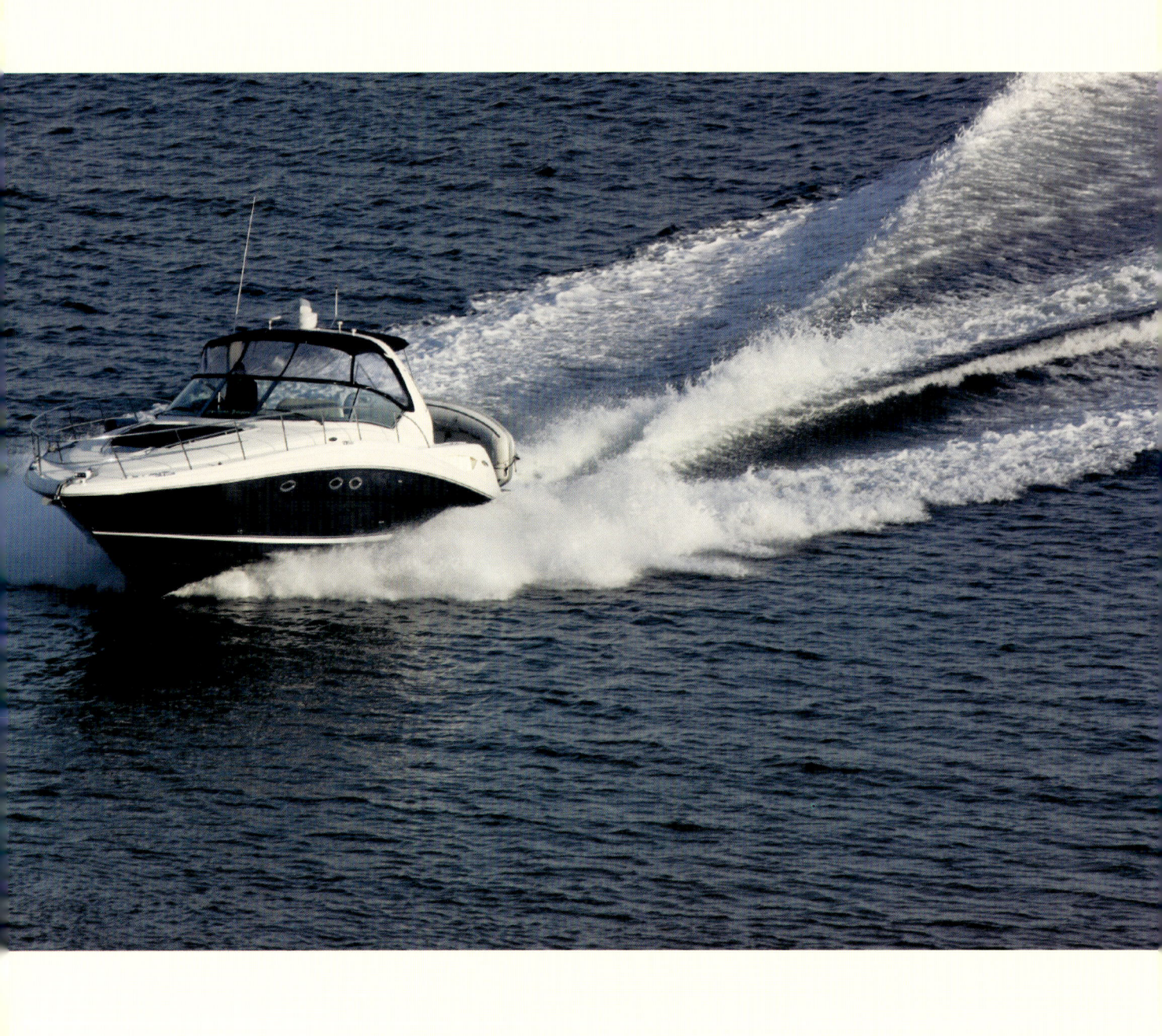

Chapter Five

I Promised Eddie I Wouldn't Send Him to a Nursing Home

Driving south on US 129, I pass Old Swimming Pool Road and Galilee Church Road. In the reservoir on the left, a speedboat churns white crests in the water. I turn off the highway and pass large newly built homes with ferns hanging from the veranda and small trailers with toys in the yard. I turn left onto an unpaved road, and the car rumbles over the gravel. A dog barks from behind a small home painted pale lime green with dark green shutters. A huge magnolia sits in the front yard, and from the backyard behind a fence, several black cows raise their heads. A trimmed hedge lines the driveway. Josephine, a tall, elegant woman with long grey hair, opens the back door and ushers me into her home.

The smell of baking fills the kitchen; a dozen brown-topped biscuits sit on a black pan on the stove. Eddie, dressed in slacks and a cotton shirt, is sitting at a small table, slowly eating his dinner of mashed potatoes, salmon croquettes, and deviled eggs. His walker sits next to his chair. A ceiling fan moves the leaves on the ivy plant hanging over the sink. As Josephine introduces me, Eddie slowly raises his left hand to signal a greeting and lifts his head slightly.

"Eddie's not much of a talker," Josephine explains. "I've been in this house forty years -- I took care of my mother and dad here. Then I started my 'extended family' -- taking people DFCS brought me. I wanted people who didn't want to be confined. It was something I wanted to do because I saw how things were going in nursing homes and I wanted people to have a home.

"Eddie had lived in some apartments in Jefferson for a good while with his mother. They'd come from Carolina I heard -- they lived on a farm. Eddie watered the horses and mules on the farm. They would get paid for picking cotton. He was born blind in one eye. I think he went to third grade. His mother died a long time ago.

"I used to see Eddie marching with the high school band down the main street of Jefferson on the Fourth of July. He must have pulled his harmonica out one day when he saw the band marching and started playing. He could blow that harmonica -- play by ear 'When the Saints Go Marching In.' One day the bandleader invited him to play solo at the Martin Luther King Day celebration at REA auditorium.

"People were taking advantage of Eddie's check and he was homeless," Josephine continues. "When DFCS brought him, he told me, 'I can cook, wash dishes, clean up. I can help you out.' Eddie used to take out the trash, feed the dogs, water the flowers -- that's before his curvature of the spine got so bad he could hardly lift his head. I got Eddie an organ and he could play songs and hymns. His favorite is 'Come by Here Good Lord, Come By Here.' Eddie would play that for Family Altar every Wednesday night at 7:00. I've done Family Altar ever since I had a family of my own. We read scripture, talked about the scripture and our problems -- helped me keep sane and take care of someone else.

"Eddie and his mother were members of New Salem Baptist -- he used to sing in the choir. Even after Eddie came to live with me he was singing in the choir. He stopped about ten years ago; it was physically too demanding. They would come and pick him up for Sunday service. Then Eddie fell and broke his hip and he couldn't go for a while."

Josephine, 73 years old and dressed in a flowing leopard-print caftan, gets up to ask Eddie if he would like some more to eat, then takes his plate to the sink. Eddie leans forward with his distinctive balding head, stands up to adjust his jeans, and sits back down. His strong jaw line leans on his chest as he listens to Josephine. "My momma had seven children and I was their momma," she says. "I went to Athens Tech -- what I need pops out when I need it. My mother and I did private duty nursing. My momma and daddy were living here when Eddie came eighteen years ago. He had a guitar then and Momma liked his music.

"When Eddie first came, he had a coffee cup in his pocket and his pants tied up with a string. He was on caffeine and hadn't been eating. My son Doug was afraid of him, but I got Eddie off caffeine, and he started eating my food, and I took him to church revival after our first meeting. I said to myself, 'If you know who Jesus is…' I was so happy. I used to get everyone up who lived here and help each one get ready for church every Sunday. How in the world did I do that?

"I take Eddie to the Senior Center and I carry him back and forth to the doctor. You don't get the right information by sending somebody else. I have never done that; I take him and will as long as I am able. One of his eyes has been blind all his life and the other one the doctor said he can't see. But I had to tell the doctor to shut up because -- I mean, you know -- your mind controls your body, and if you think you can't see, you can't, so I just told the doctor to shut up. He hushed and we came out of there because I wanted Eddie to see as long as he could see."

Eddie murmurs, "Uh huh" as Doug enters the kitchen -- a handsome man in his fifties who softly says hello to Eddie. Josephine returns from the living room, where blue flowered curtains are drawn to cool the room, with a photo album. She lifts out a picture of Eddie and three friends sitting on the couch, taken two years

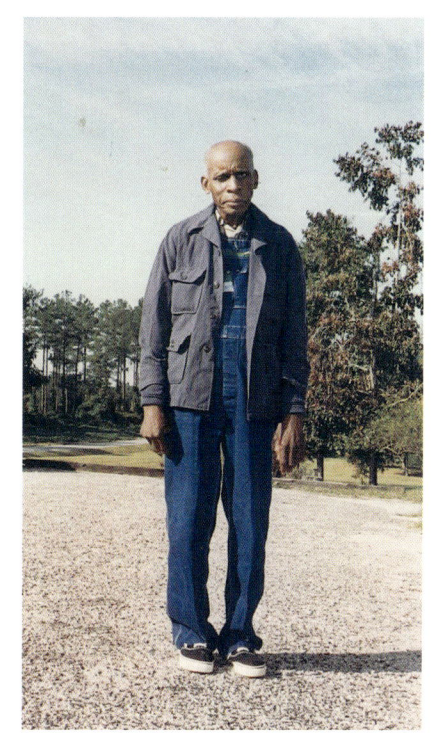

Eddie, three years after he moved in with Josephine

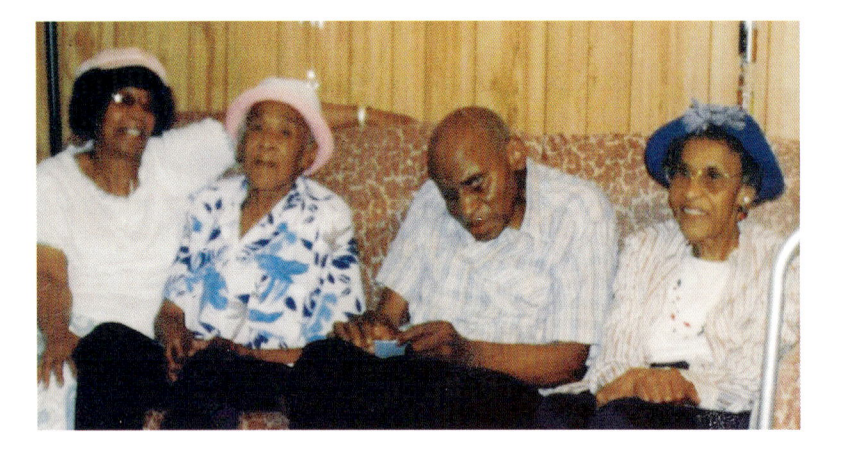

Eddie and his best friends on his 82nd birthday.

"I feel alright now I am sitting between women."

ago. Josephine tells me, "One day Doug was going to pick up Eddie's medicine. I said, 'Don't forget to give the pharmacist his birth date.' Well Doug brought home two pairs of pants, baked Eddie a cake, made him dinner. I was in church and came home and said, 'It's not Eddie's birthday yet!'"

Eddie laughs as Josephine continues, "So several weeks later on his real eighty-second birthday I invited all Eddie's friends and Doug did all the cooking: chicken wings, broccoli, and salad. We bought him an ice cream cake with a 1957 Chevrolet on it. The McDuffies came from New Salem. When we took this photo Eddie said, 'I feel alright now I am sitting between women.'"

Next to clear canisters of flour and sugar and a package of Jim Dandy grits on the counter, Doug stands at the sink, carefully cleaning the can opener. Josephine's oval face gazes proudly at her son.

"He works for the post office but he helps me out a lot!" she exclaims. "My husband used to help out too -- he was a truck driver. He died ten years ago." With wistful hazel eyes Josephine sighs, "God keeps you from getting discouraged. God called me to do what I am doing."

Josephine then asks Doug to help Eddie get ready for the revival tonight. Eddie's tall frame emerges as he rises up slowly, takes his water bottle, and with his large slender hands, moves his walker to the bathroom. Against the background of soft voices coming through the bathroom door where Doug is helping Eddie to shave, Josephine recalls, "There's revivals all around this whole month. Three Sundays ago we went up to St. Paul's Baptist near the apartments where Eddie and his mother lived. He saw a lot of people he used to know and recognized some voices. People hollered out 'Eddie!' when they saw him."

Eddie returns to the kitchen dressed in a white shirt and black suit, wearing a straw hat with a plaid hat band. He moves carefully to the family room and sits down near the back door. The room is lined with photos on floor stands of children. Pinky, a young woman in her twenties, comes through the back door with Little Man, a handsome teenager. Pinky and Little Man give Eddie a big hug and sit on the sofa.

Pinky begins, "Josephine took care of me from when I was a toddler. When I was about six, I used to get Eddie to walk with me up the pasture so I could see the cows. I would take the cows to the creek to drink. We used to go to Stone Mountain, ride the train and play in the water. Eddie was always helpful to me -- he took me outside when Josephine said 'no.'" Pinky grins at Eddie, and Eddie hums, "Uh huh."

Josephine enters the family room in a white dress with ruffles, wearing a white and black hat and smelling of perfume. With delighted surprise on her face to see Pinky and Little Man, she reminisces, "I used to take care of children at the same time -- they would always be asking Eddie, 'Do you need some water?' 'Come outside and play with me.' He would swing them, play Bingo, make up games with them."

As Pinky and Little Man hug Eddie and Josephine good bye, Josephine's large hands guide Eddie out the back door, past the wrought iron table with two chairs and a begonia pot to her car. Eddie walks slowly over the concrete and stones.

"Reach out and touch the handle of the car, turn around, and sit," Josephine reassures with her voice.

Josephine gazes at the seventy-foot magnolia tree near her car. "My mother gave me that magnolia forty years ago as a house-warming present," she says. Her fingers, painted with light pink nail polish, gesture towards Eddie, sitting in the car ready for church. "You know I admire Eddie; he is not a complainer. I slap my own self because I do complain. I can get grumpy, can't I Eddie?

"I ask God to forgive me," she continues. "It has really helped me to have somebody that needs me. It really does. I said to Eddie, 'As long as I have a place to live, you have a place to live.' So I had to keep my promise, and the only way to keep my promise was to 'adopt' him, and so that is what I did. The judge told me he never 'adopted' anyone that the mother was younger that the son! In my will it says Doug will take care of Eddie."

Then we drive over several miles and turn at a white wooden sign with a black arrow that points to "Summerhill Baptist." As Eddie emerges from the car, Josephine pulls out a wheelchair and helps Eddie sit. She pushes him up the ramp through the door and turns to seat him near the front of the small white church. Deacon Sim, dressed in a pale orange suit, greets Eddie, saying, "Hey Eddie, how are you? I heard you had a birthday this weekend. Did you dance?" Men and women dressed in suits and dresses begin to slowly walk in and find their place in one of the nine pews on either side of the church. Another deacon comes by to shake Eddie's hand; the deacons gather in front and begin to sing "Just One More Time."

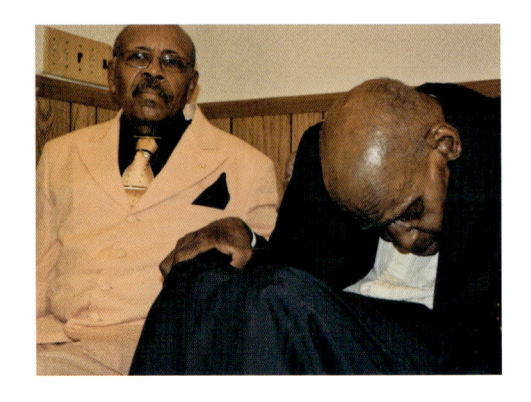

Deacon Sim and Eddie

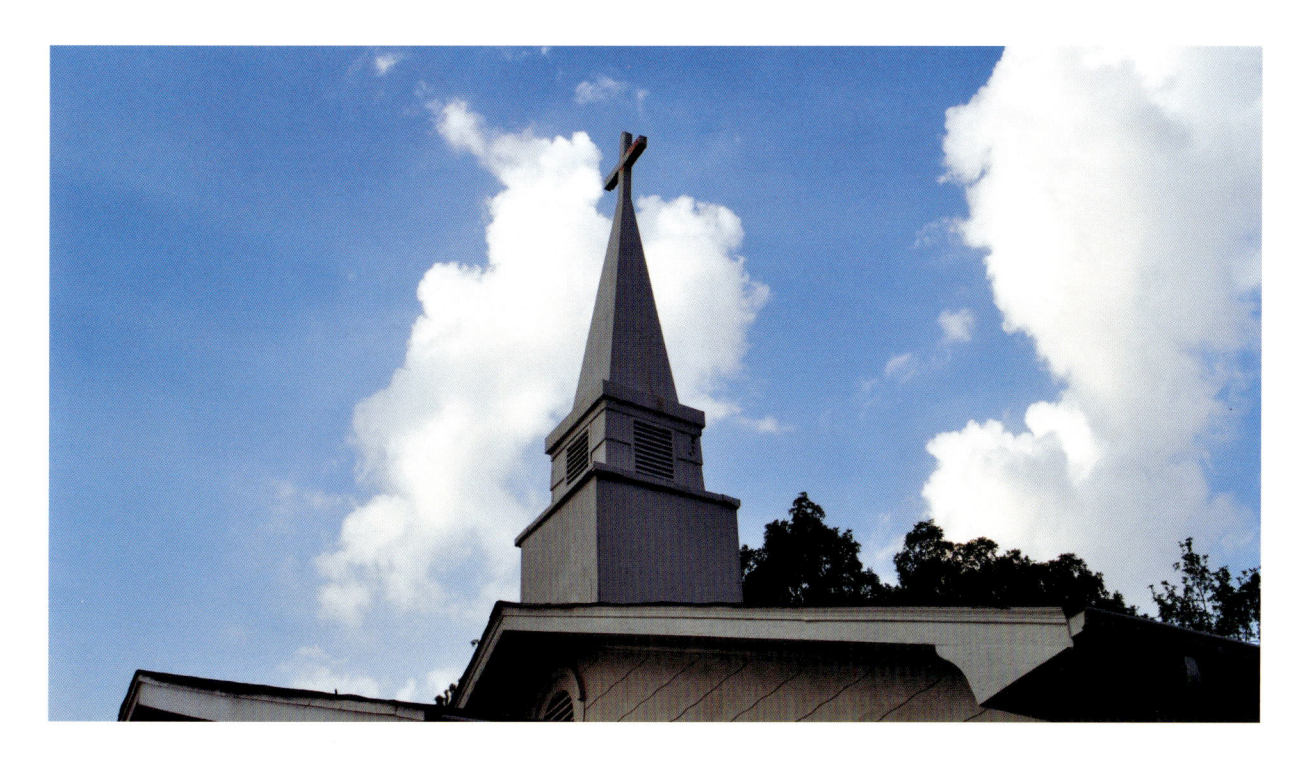

Reverend Weaver comes over to shake Eddie's hand and then sits at the organ and begins to play. One of the reverend's sons plays the drums and cymbals -- the other the guitar. As the church fills with people and music, the deacons sing "I Feel Alright in My Heart." Eddie's left foot, in his black leather shoe, taps the rhythm of the hymn on the red carpet. His hand, resting on his knee, moves up and down to the beat of the drums. Josephine takes his hand in hers, reminding him that she has kept her promise.

As the church fills with people and music, the deacons sing "I Feel Alright in My Heart."

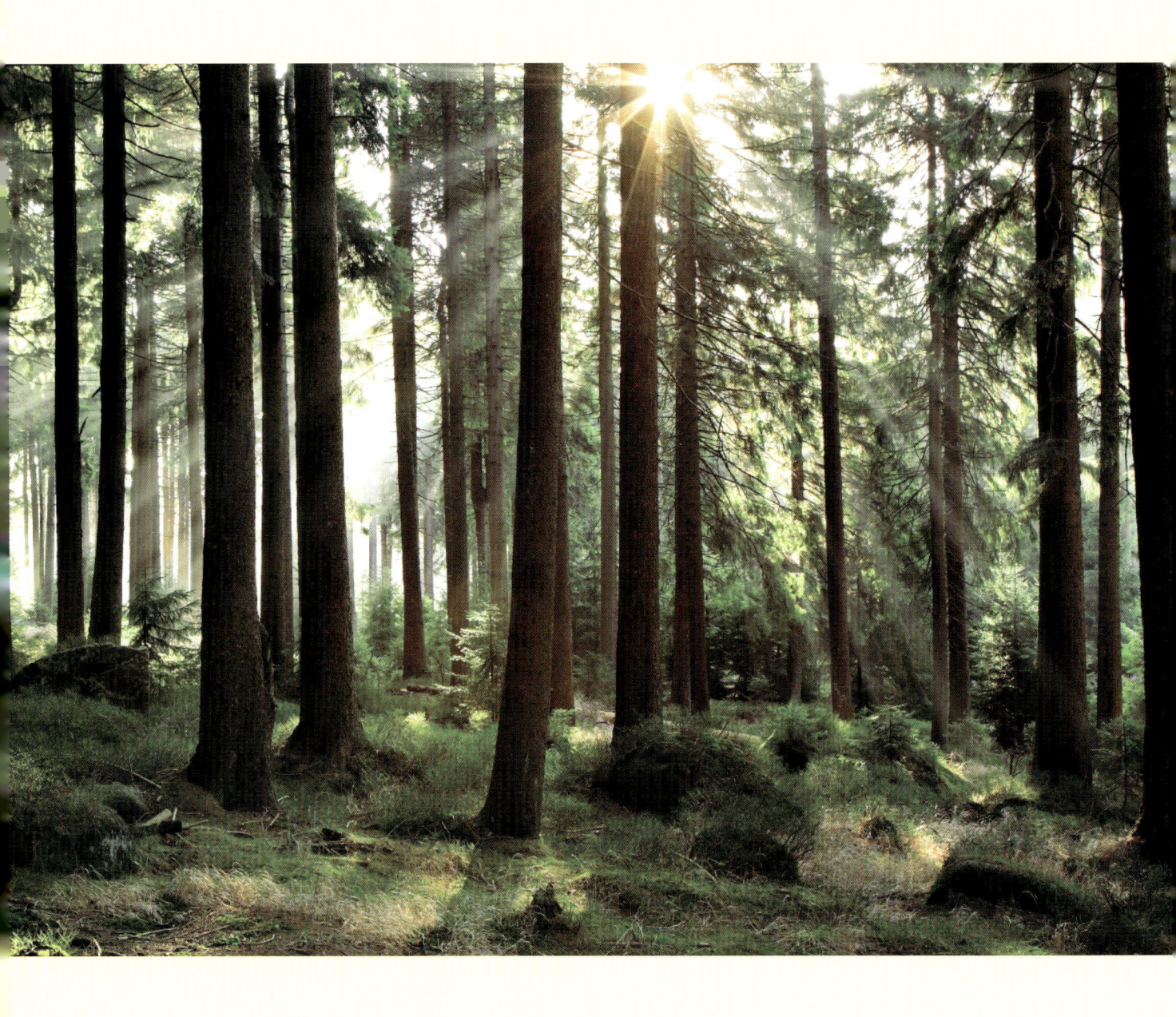

Chapter Six
Used to Go to Church Sharp As a Tack

Driving east on Georgia 72 past groves of magnificent pine trees lit from behind by the sun, I pass small signs for "peaches," "loupes," tomatoes," and "Vidalia onions" leading up to a farm stand on the right. On the left, a blue Ford V8 sits in the middle of a field, grass grown around the tires, with a "For Sale" sign peeling from inside the window. As I see barrels of hay scattered across a field and cross the Broad River, trucks begin to appear, carrying large rectangle granite chunks. I drive through the town of Elberton and turn off the four-lane into a small set of one-story apartments. I first see two red chairs, then Miss Effie, who greets me on her doorstep. Maroon dahlias, pink tea roses, and an artificial Christmas tree are all planted together in front of the window.

Effie, a slender woman of 84 years, leads me into her living room and introduces me to her sister Gennet, a handsome woman of 78 years, and Effie's daughter Winnie, who is in her fifties. We all sit on couches covered with flowered sheets and admire the walls covered with baskets and photos neatly attached with thumbtacks. Miss Effie leans forward, her face framed by short, dark grey hair and pale pink glasses, and says, "I grew up in the country -- Nickville -- had to tote water from the spring; too much rock around here. There were six of us -- just me and Gennet left. We played in the woods, hopscotch and marbles. Daddy taught me to go into the woods for home remedies.

"Gennet is named after our mother," Effie continues. "She died

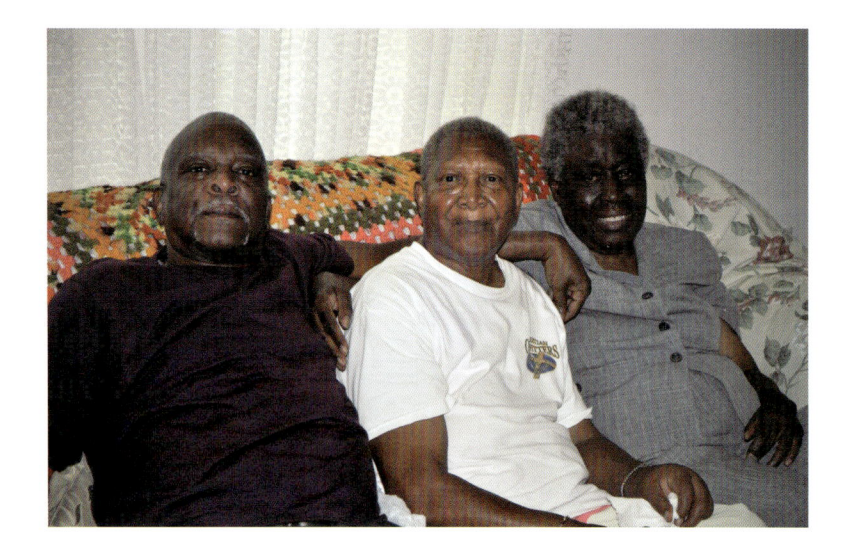

Robert, Effie and Gennet

when Gennet was two -- our father and grandmother raised us. We all walked to school eight miles; it was a one room schoolhouse on the Atlanta Highway. My daddy farmed cotton, cane, peanuts, and sweet potatoes. We raised everything we ate, and Grandmother put it up for the winter. I think she was 108 when she died -- I was sixteen then and Gennet was eleven. She was a tall dark woman with long hair who treated us good. Gennet never went to school; I left after fourth grade and worked on the farm."

Gennet, dressed in a tailored grey pantsuit, listens with intense interest as her sister describes the values under which they were raised.

"Four things carry you through the world," Effie says. "Reputation, principles, character, and manners. Got married when I was seventeen. I was hungry all the time -- my husband never came home, never brought any food. I gave what we had to eat to my six children. I wasn't weighing but seventy pounds. My Winnie -- the youngest -- they told me she wasn't going to live. Said I hadn't eaten enough to hold her. She was born premature."

Winnie, whose black hair frames her lovely face, smiles at her mother. "All of us come by to visit Mom," she says. "I come by every day for conversation." Robert Jr., Effie's son, comes through the door walking with a shiny purple cane and sits next to his mother on the couch.

Effie says, "Daddy died in 1954, and Gennet was left with my stepmother. I had to go get her -- no one would see about her. Had no help from my brother or sisters. Daddy had asked me if anything happened to him would I take care of Gennet. Back then my sister couldn't control herself with cussing. I was the only one close to my Daddy. He loved Gennet. I could hardly take care of myself but I took her. I am her sister I'm supposed to take care of her. She could have been me. After fifty-seven years, if she had been with someone else they might have been mean to her. I love my sister.

"By then my oldest boy Robert Jr. got polio," Effie continues, "and I had to tote him around on my back until he was fourteen years old. He was in an iron lung. I went back and forth to the hospital for five years. He was the first one in Elbert County to catch polio -- the doctor didn't even know what it was. I didn't let Robert Jr. miss a doctor's appointment in seventeen years. One day at the train station in Atlanta a woman looked at us as we was going up the steps. Junior's foot was dragging on the ground and I asked 'Do you see any green on me?' She said, 'I'm sorry, I just see you toting that big boy.' I said, 'He can't walk.' I taught my children if you see anyone real fat don't make fun of them, you don't know the situation they are in. If you do, go look in the glass at yourself.

"I worked for doctors and lawyers to feed my family. I cooked, cleaned, took care of their children, then came home and took care of mine. One dollar for a box of clothes washed and ironed. On a morning like this I would have done three washings by now. I toted water from the spigot -- Gennet was there with me. I bathed her and kept her clothes clean, too. I had to watch her like a hawk -- if someone told Gennet to go and pick up a rock she would. I had to make sure she was okay."

Gennet picks up a trashcan and brings it to her sister so Effie can deposit her snuff. Then she shows me her blue jean pocket book, filled with notebooks and small purses. Effie's high cheek bones grace her smile at her sister.

"Robert Jr. takes us clothes shopping for Gennet," Effie says. "I get some of mine from the Salvation Army. I got some good white friends -- people I used to work for and some I raised up; they give me clothes.

"Me and Gennet used to go to White Chapel on the second Sunday, Antioch Baptist on the third Sunday, and walk to Union Grove Church about a mile away on the fourth Sunday. Didn't go nowhere on the first Sunday. Gennet and I enjoyed the hymns. We dressed sharp as a tack!" Gennet's short salt-and-pepper hair nods as Effie hums the melody of a hymn, "O precious Lord, take my hand and lead me on and let me stand… I am weak and tired…"

Then Effie continues, "When July comes each church had a revival -- there's a big dinner at the end of the week. We loved the fried chicken, apple and sweet potato pies, collards, peas, and the pinto beans was the best. Now I go to Dove Creek Baptist. Robert Jr. takes me and then comes home and stays with Gennet. She won't be still in church.

"If you look up in the morning, looks like you can take your hand and almost touch the sun. Treat people with kindness, love, and dignity. But I learned to fight," says Effie. "In 1960 my husband busted my eardrum and hit me in the stomach. I hit him with a bat -- he left after that. White lady I used to work for carried me to a doctor. He said, 'Your life ain't worth a damn, but I am going to try to save you.' They cut all the way down my stomach to remove that knot. I was in the hospital for twelve days. My children took care of themselves and Gennet -- Robert Jr. was fifteen years old then.

"Gennet started going to the adult training center in 1969. They played Bingo, walked around, and played ball. Now she's been going to the Senior Center for seven years. They have lunch there and play Bingo. They sit a lot -- don't have enough activities. And they don't sit together like I would like them to -- all white on one side and all black on the other. God put five colors on the Earth: black, white, yellow, brown, and red. Everyone is beautiful; love ain't got no color."

Effie continues with her memories. "1970 'til '77 I worked in a nursing home," she says. "I'd come up some mornings and see people on the porch saying, 'They didn't give me no breakfast yet.' It wasn't time for breakfast. When I walked by, they always followed me. I would go to the window in the kitchen door and shake my fist to the kitchen crew, and I would be plain, and they thought I was telling the crew to get them something to eat. Then I would tell them to sit at the table and they would have breakfast in a few minutes. Some people are so kind in front of people and then mean behind closed doors. You need to treat old people good. Be kind even if they are not. What goes around comes around. "

"I stopped going to church when I had to work full time – had to work two houses to get enough money to feed my family. I walked to those houses, and before I went to work, I stopped by the hospital and bathed and fed my sister and then went to work at the houses, then went back to the hospital after work to see after my sister. Sometimes I was so cold walking home in the winter, I couldn't go in the house 'cause the heat hurt me. My brother and sisters had homes – didn't never help me out. I look at how

"Precious Lord, Take My Hand"
Gospel song written by Rev. Thomas A. Dorsey
and George Nelson Allen.

Precious Lord, take my hand
Lead me on, let me stand
I am tired, I am weak, I am worn
Through the storm, through the night
Lead me on to the light
Take my hand precious Lord,
lead me home

When my way grows drear
Precious Lord linger near
When my life is almost gone
Hear my cry, hear my call
Hold my hand lest I fall
Take my hand precious Lord,
lead me home

When the darkness appears
And the night draws near
And the day is past and gone
At the river I stand
Guide my feet, hold my hand
Take my hand precious Lord,
lead me home

Precious Lord, take my hand
Lead me on, let me stand
I'm tired, I'm weak, I'm lone
Through the storm, through the night
Lead me on to the light
Take my hand precious Lord,
lead me home

people are ashamed of people sometimes. I picked cotton to get my babies milk. After my children were grown, in 1977 I worked in the poultry plant cutting, deboning, and packing boxes. I drove to the poultry plant six miles away. Got sick in 1987 and haven't worked since then, even though I've used my home remedies.

Gennet smiles broadly as her sister continues, "The home health aid comes by every morning from 7:00-10:00 to help Gennet dress and bathe -- we've had the same woman for five years. She comes in laughing and goes out laughing. You know if someone brings joy into your house the joy stays all day. She treats my sister so good and talks to her so good -- that makes me and Gennet so happy."

Robert Jr. sits next to his mother wearing a purple shirt, his white hair and mustache distinguishing his face. "Gennet was always part of the crew, just like our older sister. I worked in the granite shed crating rock for twenty-seven years. Now that I am retired I come by every day. Sometimes we go riding, stop and talk to old friends from the car, get the boredom out of our bodies. We'll be here -- you know we just don't like to talk about who is going first."

As Effie leads me to the door, Gennet gets up and brings me a cup I have left on the table. She says goodbye with her infectious smile, and Effie picks one of her dahlias as we step outside and hands it to me. Standing next to the bright red chairs, Effie sighs, "I hadn't had no easy life. I had a hard life. Give the glory to God."

"You know if someone brings joy into your house - the joy stays all day."

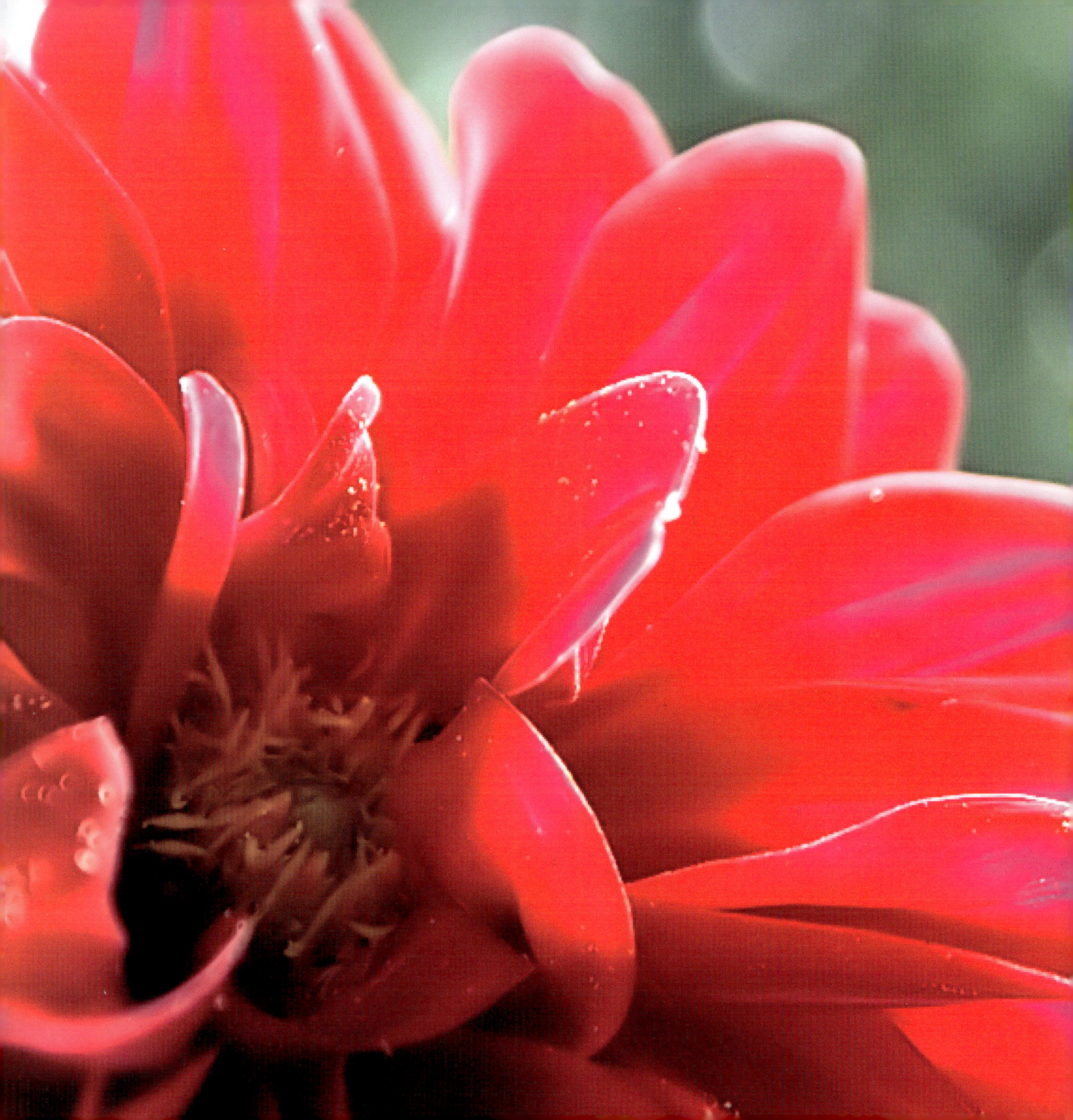

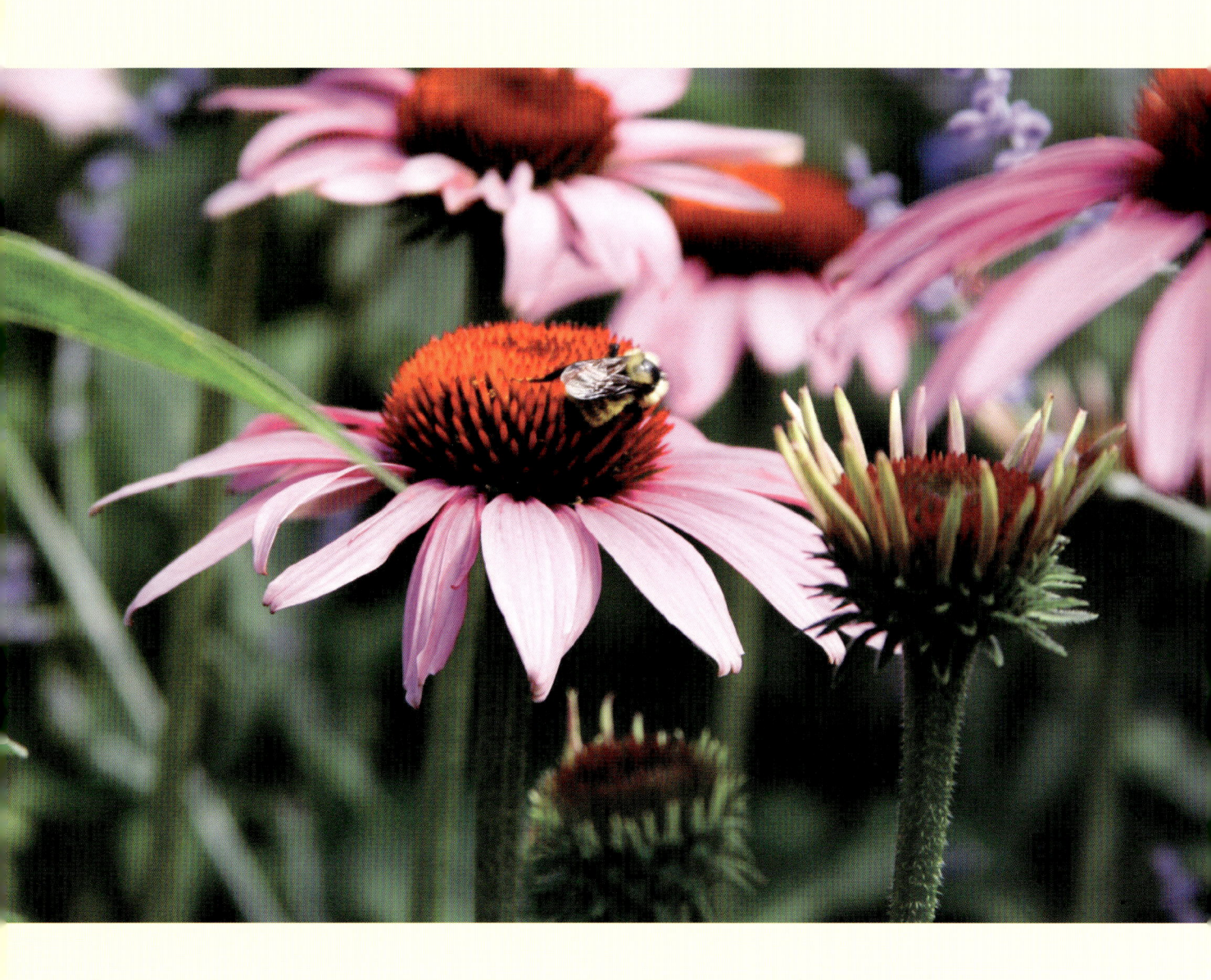

Chapter Seven

I Always Measured My Boyfriends by How They Reacted to Jimmy

Driving east on Highway 78 toward Athens, sunlight like a thousand pieces of mirrors shimmers on a pond in a nearby field. In the median strip, the pale gold bloom of tall grasses picks up the wind, and dark green kudzu covers the banks along side of the highway in mysterious shapes. Driving into Athens, I turn off a winding road into a quiet neighborhood and stop in front of a red brick home with lavender coneflowers in front. Madge, a petite woman in her fifties, greets me underneath the American flag hanging next to the front door. She shows me a seat at the large oval dining room table covered with a cotton yellow brocade tablecloth and introduces her mother Eliane, who is 90, and her brother Jimmy, who is 52.

Eliane smiles with soft blue eyes through her large glasses. "I grew up in a banlieu of Paris and moved to the United States in 1945 with my mother," she says. "She had lived in Atlanta and married a Frenchman before moving to Paris. While I was in nursing school at Emory University I met my husband who was studying to be a veterinarian at the University of Georgia." Eliane looks at her son Jimmy, a short, handsome man with brown eyes rimmed in blue. "We first lived in Lexington, Georgia -- my husband was a state veterinarian. Jimmy was born in Lexington. Some family members said to send him to an institution."

Madge, with beautiful short hair that graces her chin line, gazes at Jimmy. "You didn't see kids with Down syndrome then -- people would stop in their tracks and stare. I knew Jimmy was different, but I couldn't figure out why they were staring. I was more mad -- my older brother Joe was more embarrassed. The kids staring didn't bother me as much as the adults. I hated it," Madge recalls with tears in her blue eyes.

Eliane reaches back in her memory over 50 years. "We moved to Athens when Jimmy was two and met more families," she recalls. "When we went downtown on Clayton Street, everyone we met waved at Jimmy. Jimmy would put out his hand and say, 'Hello, my name is Jimmy.' Where we went Jimmy went -- we used to shop at Davison's and Jimmy would climb in the storefront window to hide from Mom. He would laugh when she called his name frantically looking for him. Most of the time, she had to climb in the window to get him, but he had the attention of the passersby."

Madge then recalls growing up:
"We rented a cottage every year in New Smyrna Beach, Florida for two weeks. Dad and Mom went deep-sea fishing, and we kids played with other kids nearby. Mom liked to bake red snapper and make boiled or mashed potatoes. Jimmy is the potato man. Here at home in Athens we used to go to bulldog games."

Jimmy shows me the Georgia bulldog watch he is wearing and says, "I like the red to make a touchdown and kick the ball."

"We used to go to Atlanta and visit my mother's mother, our grandmother MeMe. She worked at Western Union and wore headphones. I remember we would go downtown to Rich's and buy a chocolate cake -- Jimmy's favorite. MeMe came to visit us on the weekends. She rode the Greyhound bus to Athens. She always brought us candy. When MeMe got glaucoma she came to live with us. Jimmy was nine years old then."

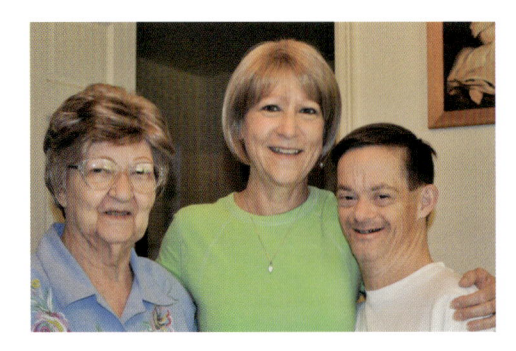

Eliane, Madge, and Jimmy

Jimmy walks me across the living room, lined with prints of the Eiffel Tower and L'Arc de Triomphe, to a small room -- a wood-lined study. On a square table sit 50 or more springs Jimmy has carefully arranged in a maze. On another table, green and black pill bottles are arranged in a pattern. He picks up a tin box, and we return to the dining room table.

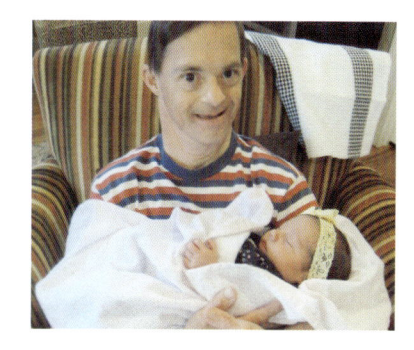

Jimmy opens the box and very gently picks up a few of the stacks of pictures of women that he has cut out from catalogues in perfect rectangles. Madge smiles with pride at her brother, saying, "Jimmy loves to work with his hands. He loved doing piecework at the sheltered workshop -- he counted out artificial worms to put in packages for a bait shop. Now the staff takes him to volunteer at the food bank and the animal shelter. He's gone to the same center since he was a pre-schooler."

Jimmy and Eden Eliane

Madge brings in a photo framed in black wood of Jimmy proudly holding his great-niece, Eden Eliane, sleeping in his lap. "Jimmy loves ceremonies," she says. "When Eden Eliane's mother Jennifer was married, she and her husband drove away in a horse and carriage. Jimmy cried at the wedding -- he would love to be married. Ceremonies fascinate Jimmy.

"On his fiftieth birthday, Jennifer put a blow up hula girl in the front yard, and we all stood waiting for the limo we had hired as a surprise -- me, Mama, our niece, Jennifer, and her husband, Joseph, our nephew, our brother, Joe, and his wife. The limo pulled up and Jimmy turned to us with his eyebrows raised: 'Me?' Jennifer had plastic wine glasses and we all toasted Jimmy with sparkling Martnelli's. We pulled up in a black limo in front of Red Lobster, Jimmy's favorite place.

"Our dad had Alzheimer's disease. We went to visit him every Sunday. Jimmy would hold his hand and tell Pop he loved him. As Pop got sicker, Jimmy became very anxious -- he can feel when something is not right. He died fourteen years ago. I can still see Jimmy standing at the funeral next to a family he used to bowl with… and hugging them," Madge sighs as a tear rolls down her cheek.

She continues, "Jimmy's name came up on the waiting list for a church group home after Daddy died, but Jimmy had lost so much weight while Dad was ill it wouldn't have been good for him to go then.

"When I was growing up," she says, "I remember tricks Jimmy used to play. Mom and Dad put a safety lock on the porch latch -- Jimmy got a broom, flipped the latch, and ran to the neighbor's house to hide. He laughed as he heard them looking for him. Then one of my friends brought Jimmy to a college sorority dance-a-thon we were attending -- when she turned her back, Jimmy was gone. She looked up and saw him on the upper floor balcony grinning at her.

"When I retired from the school system five years ago, Jimmy came to the party. When they called my name, Jimmy stood up, clapped his hands and yelled, 'Good job Madge!'

"I would come every morning to help get Jimmy ready to go to the workshop. I saw it coming with Mama -- she fell three times last year and wound up in the hospital. I moved in last November. This is my life now," Madge reflects with moistened eyes. "I still visit my house and take some time in the afternoon to do my things. I have a book club and I am helping a friend renovate his house. But I make sure the dinner is made here every day. When it's time for supper I say to Jimmy, 'Let's get married,' and we walk from here to the kitchen arm in arm singing 'Going to the Chapel of Love.' Jimmy says, 'Thank you very much Bonjour.'

"The fact that I am retired makes it okay. Had this happened when

I was working it wouldn't have been easy. What concerns me is the trustworthiness of people -- if we have to hire someone to come in and help," Madge says as she looks at her mother and Jimmy.

"Most of my good friends have gone to God -- thank the Lord Madge is willing to help," Eliane says as she blows her nose on a handkerchief edged with lace. Eliane looks with fondness at her son. "Jimmy just loves people -- the loving part is always there."

Jimmy's clean-shaven face leans close with interest as Madge describes the rodeo they attended. "Someone gave Jimmy a microphone and he sang 'God Bless America.' He loves the spotlight. When I was a kid I loved to play with Jimmy; even now my close friends from college come around, and if Jimmy is not here they say tell him I said hello. We love it when Eden Eliane comes to visit, and sometimes my brother Joe takes Jimmy fishing at lakes near Atlanta where he works. I am trying to get Joe to come more often.

"Jimmy is very intuitive and recognizes when I don't set a place for myself at the table" Madge continues. "He asks, 'Where you going?' Jimmy is sweet, obstinate, loving, funny, loud, caring, and he's Jimmy. If my friends hadn't liked Jimmy… they weren't my friends. I always measured my boyfriends by how they reacted to Jimmy," she says softly as tears roll down her cheek, revealing the depth of her fidelity to her family.

"Jimmy is sweet, obstinate, loving, funny, loud, caring, and he's Jimmy."

I come, in conclusion, to the difference between 'projecting' the future and making a promise. The 'projecting' of 'futurologists' uses the future as the safest possible context for whatever is desired, it binds me only to selfish intent. But making a promise binds one to someone else's future. If the promise is serious enough, one is brought to it by love and in awe and fear. Fear, awe, and love bind us to no selfish aims but to each other. And they enforce a speech more exact, more clarifying, and more binding than any speech that can be used to sell or advocate some 'future.' For when we promise in love and awe and fear there is a certain kind of mobility that we give up. We give up the romance of program that is always shifting its terms to fit its occasions. We are speaking where we stand, and we shall stand afterwards in the presence of what we have said

Wendell Berry,
Standing by Words